Dear Doctor:

Fast Facts—Irritable Bowel Syndrome
has been provided as a service to your
medical practice. The information presented
reflects the knowledge of experts in their
respective fields on a disease that affects
your practice every day.

It has been provided to you
with compliments from Eisai Inc. and
Janssen Pharmaceutica Inc.

Accept this with our thanks.

Sincerely,
Eisai Inc. and Janssen Pharmaceutica Inc.

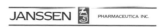

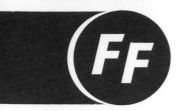

FAST FACTS

Indispensable Guides to Clinical Practice

Irritable Bowel Syndrome

Second edition

W Grant Thompson
Former Consultant Gastroenterologist,
Ottawa Hospital,
and Emeritus Professor of Medicine,
University of Ottawa, Ontario, Canada

Kenneth W Heaton
Former Consultant Physician,
Bristol Royal Infirmary,
and Doctor of Science,
University of Bristol, UK

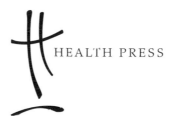

HEALTH PRESS

Oxford

© Health Press 2003
This local reprint of *Fast Facts–Irritable Bowel Syndrome, Second Edition* is published by arrangement with Health Press Limited.

Fast Facts – Irritable Bowel Syndrome
First published 1999 as Fast Facts – Irritable Bowel Syndrome by Kenneth W Heaton and W Grant Thompson
Second edition April 2003
Text © 2003 W Grant Thompson, Kenneth W Heaton

© 2003 in this edition Health Press Limited
Health Press Limited, Elizabeth House, Queen Street, Abingdon, Oxford OX14 3JR, UK
Tel: +44 (0)1235 523233
Fax: +44 (0)1235 523238

Fast Facts is a trade mark of Health Press Limited.

A CIP catalogue record for this title is available from the British Library.

ISBN 1-903734-33-9

Thompson, WG (W Grant)
Fast Facts – Irritable Bowel Syndrome/
W Grant Thompson, Kenneth W Heaton

Illustrated by Gillian Lee Illustrations, Buckhurst Hill, UK.
Typesetting and page layout by Zed, Oxford, UK.
Printed in the United States of America

This book has been printed using vegetable inks and paper manufactured from sustainable forests, and is fully biodegradable and recyclable.

Foreword

George F Longstreth, MD
Chief of Gastroenterology, Kaiser Permanente Medical Center, San Diego, California

In this revision of *Fast Facts – Irritable Bowel Syndrome*, Drs W Grant Thompson and Kenneth W Heaton have updated their comprehensive, concise and useful practice guide on the management of patients with IBS. The additional information will help practitioners care for patients with this common cause of abdominal pain and bowel habit abnormality.

The authors include recent developments in pathophysiology, diagnosis and treatment in a readable style that combines objectivity with the wisdom of experience. Potentially important processes in the central nervous system and the gut are described, including evidence of mucosal inflammation that even challenges the traditional classification of IBS as a 'functional' disorder. However, the authors emphasize the difficulty of distinguishing the causality of observed pathophysiological correlates from epiphenomena. On a background of their research on the Manning symptom criteria 25 years ago and their subsequent work on periodic diagnostic criteria revisions, most recently the Rome II criteria, they discuss what is currently known about the comparability of the various diagnostic criteria. Their detailed tips on history taking and interacting with patients, including how to elicit psychological factors and explain them, are especially valuable to both general and specialist practitioners. Economy is served by their advice that a diagnosis in most patients can be based on the presence of typical symptoms, the absence of alarm symptoms, and limited testing. Their assessment of the new, promising serotonergic neuroenteric modulators is accurate and appropriately balanced with skepticism regarding the value of any single drug for a disorder with such a diverse pathophysiological and clinical spectrum. Above all, these respected clinicians emphasize that 'the doctor is the placebo', an often neglected concept that has great potential therapeutic value.

When Drs Thompson and Heaton began their professional careers, they likely could have flipped through month after month of

5

gastroenterology journals before finding an article on IBS. Nowadays, not only is the disorder emerging from such darkness, but the proliferating publication of laboratory research, clinical observations, subject reviews, consensus documents and sophisticated mathematical applications (e.g. meta-analyses) can bewilder a practitioner who primarily wants to know how to diagnose and treat patients. This guide to clinical practice fulfills this need well.

Introduction

This book is the fruit of a transatlantic collaboration spanning 25 years and culminating in a research project based on general practices in the Bristol area of England. When we wrote our first paper together, few people were interested in irritable bowel syndrome (IBS) but, since then, it has become the subject of much scientific inquiry (Figure 1) and also one of great public interest. Much has been learned about its clinical features, its diagnosis and, in particular, its epidemiology.

We now know that IBS is the most common explanation for gut symptoms in the community, the most common reason that people go to their family doctor with a gut complaint and the most common

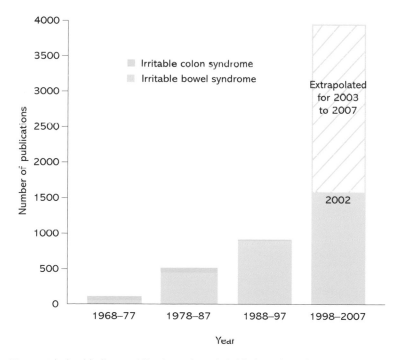

Figure 1 Index Medicus publications about irritable bowel syndrome, or irritable colon syndrome as it used to be called, in the decade before and in the decades after 1978. This was the year in which the authors described the symptoms that enable a positive diagnosis to be made (now known as the 'Manning criteria').

diagnosis in patients who are referred to a gastroenterologist. Despite all this, specialists are still groping to understand the pathogenesis of IBS, and it is a rash doctor who claims to cure it once and for all.

IBS presents itself to the world in many guises. Not only do symptoms vary between patients, but also a single patient's symptoms vary over time. In addition, IBS is perceived differently by patients and non-patients, that is to say people who have the symptoms but do not complain about them. It is seen differently again by each of the many groups of healthcare workers who become involved – family physicians, gastroenterologists, internists, surgeons, gynecologists, psychologists, psychiatrists and healthcare managers. Perhaps because of these varied perspectives, a plethora of belief systems has grown up about the nature of IBS, and we believe that none of them is likely to be wholly true.

In the first edition of *Fast Facts – Irritable Bowel Syndrome*, we attempted to present the scientific facts about IBS clearly and impartially. We also built on our personal experience in proposing a management approach that we believe is a practical and sensible one for family physicians and for other doctors. In the four years since the first edition was published, significant developments have occurred which convinced us of the need to add to and update the book. New epidemiological studies have extended our knowledge of IBS worldwide, and notions that visceral sensitivity or occult inflammation may lie behind the syndrome have been further explored. Experience with diagnostic criteria has grown, and the case for an economical approach to investigations has been strengthened. Patient support groups and pharmaceutical companies have raised the public profile of IBS and promoted new research. For the first time, well-designed trials have shown benefit from drugs and psychological therapy, at least for selected patients. Of course, new data raise new questions, and we discuss these at the end of this book. Unfortunately, management of IBS continues to be handicapped by our ignorance of its pathogenesis and by obstacles in healthcare systems to the nurturing of the all-important doctor–patient relationship, the traditional virtues of which, we steadfastly believe, hold the keys to successful management. Nevertheless there is progress and much to be optimistic about.

1 What is IBS?

Irritable bowel syndrome (IBS) is a constellation of symptoms that doctors recognize when taking a medical history. The symptoms appear to be due to dysfunction of the intestine and are said, therefore, to be 'functional'. They consist of abdominal pain related to defecation, altered bowel habit and – variably – other symptoms such as abdominal bloating or visible distension, a feeling of incomplete evacuation, and mucus in the stools. Typically the bowel habit is chaotic – sometimes 'normal', sometimes constipation, sometimes diarrhea, sometimes both extremes in the same day.

Unlike a structural or 'organic' disease, such as peptic ulcer, there is no anatomical lesion that explains the symptoms and that, when found, clinches the diagnosis. There is not even a clear-cut pathophysiological explanation. While the patient's gut is clearly malfunctioning, current technology cannot precisely measure the abnormality, nor can any test assist the doctor in making the diagnosis.

Hence, we know of the existence of IBS only from patients' descriptions of their symptoms. The challenge for the doctor is to recognize the pattern of symptoms that identifies IBS. Our ability to do this began with a study carried out by the authors back in 1977–78. We administered questionnaires to patients referred by GPs to medical and surgical clinics in Bristol and found that six symptoms were more prevalent in IBS than in organic abdominal disease. These became known as the 'Manning criteria' (Table 1.1). The more that were present, the more likely was it that the patient had IBS (Figure 1.1). These symptom criteria have been validated by others and are used worldwide in epidemiological studies, clinical trials and everyday practice.

In recent years teams of experts, meeting in Rome and using a consensus approach, have developed definitions and symptom criteria for all the recognized functional gastrointestinal disorders (Table 1.2). It is a formidable list and only specialists make many of the diagnoses, but it is important for family doctors and generalists to know that these

TABLE 1.1

Manning criteria for IBS

By convention, a diagnosis of IBS requires abdominal pain and at least two of the following six criteria. The first three are the basis for the Rome II criteria (Table 1.4).

- Abdominal pain eased after bowel movement
- Looser stools at onset of pain
- More frequent bowel movements at onset of pain
- Abdominal distension
- Mucus per rectum
- Feeling of incomplete emptying

Source: Manning et al. 1978

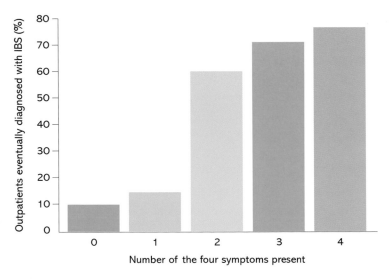

Figure 1.1 Percentage of patients diagnosed as having IBS on referral to hospital clinics with abdominal pain or disturbed bowel habits, according to how many of four symptoms they admitted to at their first clinic visit. The four symptoms were relief of pain with defecation, looser stools since onset of pain, more frequent stools since onset of pain, and abdominal distension (the first three are the Rome II criteria). These symptoms later became incorporated into the Manning criteria, together with feelings of incomplete evacuation and passage of mucus.

TABLE 1.2

The functional gastrointestinal disorders*

Functional esophageal disorders

- Globus
- Rumination syndrome
- Functional chest pain of presumed esophageal origin
- Functional heartburn
- Functional dysphagia
- Unspecified functional esophageal disorder

Functional gastroduodenal disorders

- Functional dyspepsia[†]
- Ulcer-like dyspepsia
- Dysmotility-like dyspepsia
- Unspecified (non-specific) dyspepsia
- Aerophagia
- Functional vomiting

Functional bowel disorders

- Irritable bowel syndrome
- Functional abdominal bloating[†]
- Functional constipation[†]
- Functional diarrhea[†]
- Unspecified functional bowel disorder

Functional abdominal pain

- Functional abdominal pain syndrome[†]
- Unspecified functional abdominal pain

Functional disorders of the biliary tract and pancreas

- Gallbladder dysfunction
- Sphincter of Oddi dysfunction

Functional anorectal disorders

- Functional fecal incontinence
- Functional anorectal pain
- Levator syndrome
- Proctalgia fugax
- Pelvic floor dyssynergia
- Unspecified functional anorectal disorder

* Some experts are now calling functional gastrointestinal disorders 'disorders of gastrointestinal function'
[†] IBS should be distinguished from functional abdominal bloating, functional constipation, functional diarrhea, functional dyspepsia and functional abdominal pain because these present different diagnostic and treatment issues
Source: Drossman et al. 2000

other gut disorders exist because some of them overlap with IBS. Moreover, each has its own diagnostic and therapeutic challenges. In this book we concentrate on IBS, the commonest and most studied of the functional gastrointestinal disorders, but we shall make brief reference to five others because they are sometimes confused with IBS:

- abdominal bloating
- functional constipation
- functional diarrhea
- functional dyspepsia
- functional abdominal pain syndrome (FAPS).

Relevant definitions are shown in Table 1.3. The current diagnostic criteria for IBS (Rome II criteria) are based on the Manning criteria and

TABLE 1.3

Definitions relevant to IBS

Functional gastrointestinal disorder (disorder of gastrointestinal function)

- Chronic or recurrent gastrointestinal symptoms not explained by structural or biochemical abnormalities (symptoms may be attributable to any level of the gastrointestinal tract from oropharynx to anus)

Functional bowel disorder

- A functional gastrointestinal disorder with symptoms attributable to the mid or lower intestinal tract

Irritable bowel syndrome

- A functional bowel disorder in which abdominal pain is associated with defecation or a change in bowel habit, usually with features of disordered defecation and with distension

Functional abdominal pain syndrome (also called chronic idiopathic abdominal pain or chronic functional abdominal pain)

- Abdominal pain for at least 6 months with loss of daily functioning, the pain being unrelated to physiological activity in the gut and unexplained by structural or other functional gastrointestinal disorder

After Thompson et al. 1999

TABLE 1.4

Diagnostic criteria* for IBS (the 'Rome II criteria')

Twelve weeks[†] or more in the past 12 months of abdominal discomfort or pain that has two of the following three features, in the absence of structural or metabolic abnormalities to explain the symptoms:

- relief with defecation
- association with a change in frequency of stool
- association with a change in form (appearance) of stool

One or more of the following symptoms, on at least a quarter of occasions or days, is usually present, and may be used to identify different sub-groups of IBS. They are not essential for diagnosis, but add to the doctor's confidence that the intestine is the source of the abdominal pain. The more symptoms that are present, the more confident the diagnosis:

- abnormal stool frequency (> 3/day or < 3/week)
- abnormal stool form (lumpy/hard or loose/watery)
- abnormal stool passage (straining, urgency or feeling of incomplete evacuation)
- passage of mucus
- bloating or feeling of abdominal distension

* See Table 4.2, page 38, for questions designed to elicit these symptoms
[†] It is not necessary for the 12 weeks to be consecutive. For clinical or survey use, the period is modified to 'the last 3 months'
After Thompson et al. 1999

are shown in Table 1.4. Like their predecessors, the Rome I criteria, they were generated using a consensus procedure by an international team of gastroenterologists with a special interest in functional disorders. They were designed for research purposes, but they are of practical value to clinicians, assisting them to recognize the essential features of IBS and to diagnose it with confidence (Chapter 4, Diagnosis). As the next chapter will indicate, IBS itself is a huge problem in terms of prevalence, but it need not be a problem to diagnose. We believe it can be confidently identified through a careful history, the diagnostic criteria we have mentioned, and appropriate questioning and physical examination. Family doctors can safely diagnose IBS with few, if any, tests, particularly in younger adults. Positive and confident diagnosis is a central theme of this book.

What is IBS? – Key points

- IBS is the commonest and best studied of many functional gastrointestinal disorders.
- Its diagnosis depends upon symptoms, currently the Rome II criteria.
- Alarm symptoms are not due to IBS and should provoke further enquiry.

Key references

Camilleri M, Choi M-G. Irritable bowel syndrome (Review). *Aliment Pharmacol Ther* 1997;11:3–15.

Drossman DA, Corazziari E, Talley NJ, et al. *The Functional Gastrointestinal Disorders*, 2nd edn. McLean (VA): Degnon, 2000.

Heaton KW. Irritable bowel syndrome. In: Bouchier IAD, Allan RN, Hodgson HJF, Keighley MRB, eds. *Gastroenterology: Clinical Science and Practice*, 2nd edn. London: WB Saunders, 1993:1512–22.

Manning AP, Thompson WG, Heaton KW et al. Towards positive diagnosis of the irritable bowel. *BMJ* 1978;2:653–4.

Thompson WG. The irritable bowel syndrome: pathogenesis and management. *Lancet* 1993;341: 1569–72.

Thompson WG, Longstreth GF, Drossman DA et al. Functional bowel disorders and functional abdominal pain. *Gut* 1999;45 (suppl II):II43–7.

Zighelboim J, Talley NJ. What are functional bowel disorders? *Gastroenterology* 1993;104: 1196–201.

The individual symptoms of IBS are so common in the community that one could argue they are part of the human condition. Scarcely any adult would deny that he or she has experienced at some time abdominal cramps, altered bowel habit or feelings of abdominal distension. However, when the symptoms come together as a cluster, become persistent or interfere with work and leisure, they must be judged abnormal, that is, a disease. Of course, IBS is not a mortal disease, but it is seldom cured, coming and going throughout life.

Historical perspective

Irritable bowel syndrome is not a disease of modern living. It was amply described in the 19th century. However, its nature may have changed over the years. For example, older accounts placed emphasis on rectal discharge of mucus but this phenomenon is seldom complained of nowadays. The first systematic account of the syndrome was in a classic 1962 paper by Chaudhary and Truelove. That paper was entitled 'The Irritable Colon', but we now believe that more than the colon is involved. In English, the term *irritable bowel* replaced *irritable colon* in the 1970s but, in French and Spanish, the term *colon* persists (*le côlon irritable* and *sindrome de colon irritable*).

International studies

The authors' collaboration began in 1977 when, suspecting IBS to be very prevalent in the community, we interviewed 301 apparently healthy English people about their bowel habits and symptoms. Fourteen percent admitted to symptoms consistent with IBS (Figure 2.1). Subsequent surveys in the USA, France, New Zealand and elsewhere produced similar findings, establishing that IBS is very common worldwide. In these studies, only a third to a half of those with diagnosable IBS had seen a doctor for their complaints; in our case, only 20% had done so (Figure 2.2). A recent Canadian survey found that 13.1 % of the population had IBS using Rome I criteria and

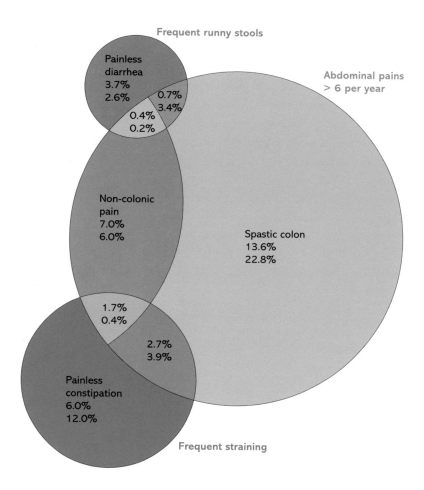

Frequent runny stools

Painless
diarrhea
3.7%
2.6%

0.7%
3.4%

0.4%
0.2%

Abdominal pains
> 6 per year

Non-colonic
pain
7.0%
6.0%

Spastic colon
13.6%
22.8%

1.7%
0.4%

2.7%
3.9%

Painless
constipation
6.0%
12.0%

Frequent straining

Figure 2.1 Data from English and Chinese studies (Thompson and Heaton 1980; Bi-Zhen and Qi-Ying 1988) showing the proportions of apparently healthy people who admit to abdominal pain and/or bowel problems and the overlap between the groups; Chinese data are those in the second row. In early studies, IBS was called 'spastic colon'.

12.1% using Rome II (Figure 2.3). However, IBS is not just a disease of 'Western' countries. It has been reported to be common in Africa and Asia, while surveys in China and Bangladesh have yielded results remarkably similar to ours in England (Figure 2.1). Thus it seems that IBS troubles humanity everywhere.

Gender differences

In most population surveys, the prevalence of IBS is twice as great in women as in men. In hospital clinics, the female to male ratio is even higher (Table 2.1). In English general practice, 86% of IBS patients are female. It seems, therefore, that not only do more females than males experience IBS, but also that, once they have the symptoms, women are more likely to consult a doctor about them. It is important to realize that having symptoms is not the only factor in an IBS sufferer's decision to see a doctor. Cultural factors are probably involved since, in India, Sri Lanka and Japan, men are more likely than women to report the disease (Table 2.1).

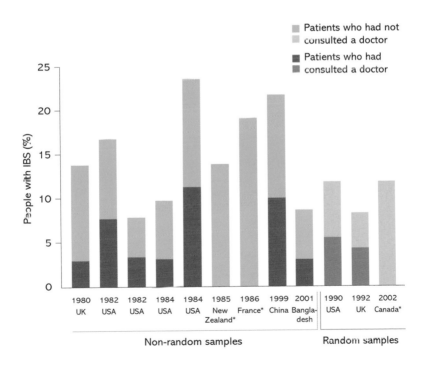

Figure 2.2 Prevalence of IBS in apparently healthy populations, and the proportion of those with IBS who had consulted a doctor. IBS was usually defined as recurrent abdominal pain relieved by defecation. * Doctor consultation data not available.

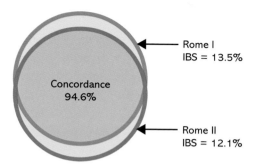

Figure 2.3 Prospective application of the Rome I and Rome II criteria to a random telephone sample of 1100 Canadian adults. These two sets of criteria identify similar individuals with a high degree of agreement. (The Rome II questionnaire asked: 'In the last three months did you often have discomfort or pain in your abdomen?') Source: Thompson WG et al. 2002.

TABLE 2.1

Gender distribution of IBS subjects

	Year	Location of study	Female (%)
In the general population	1992	UK	72
	1993	USA	65
	2001	Bangladesh	65
	2002	Canada	64
Consulting their family physician	1995	UK	86
Attending specialist clinics (West)	1980	UK	74
	1983	Sweden	70
	1983	UK	80
	1983	Canada	74
	1984	Canada	79
(East)	1966	New Delhi	28
	1970	Bombay	26
	1972	Raipur	18
	1982	Colombo	30

Prognosis

Irritable bowel syndrome is a chronic, yet often remitting, condition; episodes of active symptoms are followed by periods of relative inactivity. When a sample of the population is surveyed twice, a year or more apart, it is found that some people who used to have symptoms have now lost them and an equal number have acquired them. Thus, although the percentage of people with IBS may remain constant – at 17–18% – the individuals making up this figure keep changing (Figure 2.4.) It follows that, over a lifetime, the average person has a much greater than 17% chance of suffering IBS.

Unfortunately, cure is an unrealistic goal for most sufferers. We know from long-term follow-up studies that comfortingly few patients develop other gut disease and that, in those who do, the new disease is benign and unrelated to the original symptoms (Figure 2.5a). However, most patients keep having bowel symptoms (Figure 2.5b). Thus IBS patients can be told firmly that, although cure is unlikely, they will have good periods, that there are no organic complications and that there is

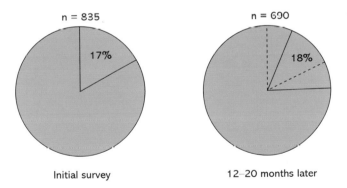

Figure 2.4 Proportion of population found to have IBS in two consecutive surveys. Seventeen percent of 835 people fulfilled IBS criteria in the first survey. Of these, 690 agreed to re-interview 12–22 months later. The point prevalence remained constant, but some of the original cohort no longer admitted symptoms while a similar number of those originally without IBS had acquired them. It follows that the lifetime risk of IBS is much greater than 17%. Source: Talley et al. 1992.

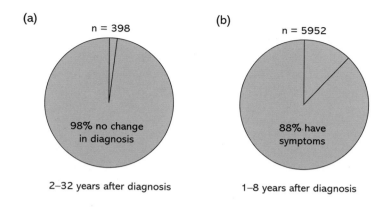

(a) n = 398

98% no change
in diagnosis

2–32 years after diagnosis

(b) n = 5952

88% have
symptoms

1–8 years after diagnosis

Figure 2.5 Prognosis of IBS: chart (a) shows that a diagnosis of IBS, when carefully made, is a safe one. Of 398 patients (in 4 studies) diagnosed with IBS, only 2% required a new gut diagnosis in the next 2–32 years. Chart (b) shows that IBS is chronic and recurring. Of almost 6000 IBS patients (from 6 studies) reviewed after 1–8 years, 88% still had gut symptoms (note: IBS criteria were not applied). Sources: Thompson 2002 and references 42–48 therein.

certainly no excess mortality. Indeed, such reassurance is an essential part of their management.

A global view
In that minority of sufferers who consult a doctor, most are likely to see only their family physician. In a survey in and around Bristol, we found that the average general practitioner, encountering eight IBS patients per week (one of whom is new), manages 70% of them without referral to a specialist. (When referrals are made their purpose is to confirm the diagnosis or to perform a test.) Thus, very few IBS sufferers get to see a specialist. Even fewer are referred on to academic centers where the possibility arises of their being entered into a clinical trial or submitted to physiological or psychological studies (Figure 2.6). Yet it is these few, highly selected patients on whom is based almost the entire body of published material about IBS.

The filtering process just described may distort people's understanding of IBS. A case in point is in the relationship of IBS to psychological disorders. Studies in academic centers consistently show much psychiatric morbidity in IBS patients, whereas surveys in the community find that non-patients with IBS are psychologically similar to the rest of the population. Patients whose IBS is managed wholly in primary care have been little studied, but they are presumably intermediate in their psychological profile. In our general practice patients, those who had been referred to a specialist were less likely than unreferred patients to recognize stress as a factor in their symptoms. Denial of stress could help explain failure to respond to their family physician's treatment.

The filtering process helps to explain a paradox. Gastroenterologists tend to consider IBS patients difficult to manage whereas (in our survey at least) family physicians perceive them as less difficult than patients with other chronic, painful and unexplained symptoms such as backache and headache. It seems likely that what prompts a minority of people with IBS to see their family physician and so become patients is their psychological status, and their disease beliefs and fears. The intransigence of these characteristics is one reason why some patients are referred on to gastroenterologists and surgeons. (This is

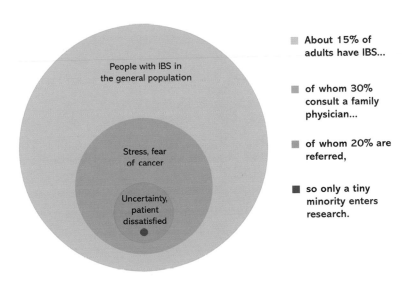

Figure 2.6 Scheme to show how IBS patients who enter research studies are highly selected and so likely to be atypical.

unfortunate, since these specialists have little training in dealing with psychosocial morbidity.)

However – and this is the point we wish to make – obtrusive though these characteristics may be, they do not necessarily tell us the origin of the problem, nor guide us as to how best to treat the majority of patients, namely, those managed wholly in primary care.

It is noteworthy that IBS constitutes up to half of the gastroenterologist's outpatient practice but only 2% of the general practitioner's caseload. The prevalence of a condition must color the physician's perception of it. All these perspectives and perceptions are relevant when designing guidelines for investigation and management.

Epidemiology – Key points

- IBS is common worldwide, especially in women.
- Most people with the syndrome do not consult doctors.
- Culture, gender and comorbidity influence the tendency to seek healthcare.
- IBS is chronic and remitting and has no serious medical consequences.

Key references

Bi-Zhen W, Qi-Ying P. Functional bowel disorders in apparently healthy Chinese people. *Chin J Epid* 1988;9: 345–9.

Chaudhary NA, Truelove SC. The irritable colon syndrome. *Q J Med* 1962;31:307–22.

Drossman DA, McKee DC, Sandler RS et al. Psychosocial factors in the irritable bowel syndrome. A multivariate study of patients and non-patients with irritable bowel syndrome. *Gastroenterology* 1988;95:701–8.

Heaton KW. Epidemiology of irritable bowel syndrome. *Eur J Gastroenterol Hepatol* 1994;6:465–9.

Kay L, Jørgensen T, Jensen KH. The epidemiology of irritable bowel syndrome in a random population:prevalence, incidence, natural history and risk factors. *J Intern Med* 1994;236:23–30.

Masud MA, Hasan M, Khan AK. Irritable bowel syndrome in a rural community in Bangladesh: prevalence, symptoms pattern, and health care seeking behavior. *Am J Gastroenterol* 2001;96:1547–52.

Talley NJ, Weaver AL, Zinsmeister AR et al. Onset and disappearance of gastrointestinal symptoms and functional gastrointestinal disorders. *Am J Epidemiol* 1992;136:165–77.

Thompson WG. Gender differences in irritable bowel symptoms. *Eur J Gastroenterol Hepatol* 1997;9: 299–302.

Thompson WG, Heaton KW. Functional bowel disorders in apparently healthy people. *Gastroenterology* 1980;79:283–8.

Thompson WG, Irvine EJ, Pare P et al. Functional gastrointestinal disorders in Canada: first population-based survey using the Rome II criteria with suggestions for improving the questionnaire. *Dig Dis Sci* 2002;47:225–35.

Thompson WG, Heaton KW, Smyth T, Smyth C. Irritable bowel syndrome in general practice: prevalence, management and referral. *Gut* 2000; 46:78–82.

Wells NEJ, Hahn BA, Whorwell PJ. Clinical economics review: irritable bowel syndrome. *Aliment Pharmacol Ther* 1997;11:1019–30.

We call IBS a disorder of gastrointestinal function, but our understanding of its pathogenesis is rudimentary. The great variability of symptoms over time makes it unlikely that it is caused by a fixed abnormality like a receptor defect, let alone a low-grade inflammatory process, as some believe. Observers' views of it depend upon their standpoint. Patients, noticing a worsening of symptoms after meals, are inclined to blame foods they have eaten. Mental health professionals, to whom patients with psychosocial morbidity are referred, understandably consider that this is where the cause lies. Gastroenterologists, who see 'difficult' patients with much comorbidity and life stresses like abuse, emphasize these features. In contrast, primary care doctors regard IBS as less troublesome than headache or backache. Epidemiologists see great numbers, economists see great costs, patient advocates see great disability and pharmaceutical companies see great markets. The many faces of IBS need reconciliation if we are to understand and manage it better.

What goes wrong in IBS and why does it go wrong? Plausible theories must be consistent with key clinical and epidemiological features of IBS. These include:

- ubiquity: bowel symptoms affect most people, certainly most women, at some time in their lives; most do not complain about them
- intermittency: IBS comes and goes, sometimes over hours or days, often over months or years
- absence of manifest pathology or pathophysiology: only symptoms mark the syndrome
- overlap with other functional symptoms, particularly from the upper gut
- less psychological morbidity in non-consulting versus consulting individuals.

A dietary disorder?

When constipation is induced using drugs in normal volunteers, they develop symptoms of IBS. This suggests that a drop in fiber intake could have the same effect. However, as a group, IBS patients eat no less fiber than other people, so fiber deficiency cannot be a major cause. Many patients blame specific foods, but organic food intolerance rather than food aversion is very hard to prove objectively. The act of eating stimulates the intestine into greater activity, a phenomenon called the 'gastrocolonic response'. Consequently, eating can induce bowel symptoms non-specifically in anyone with a tendency that way. In IBS, this may be particularly likely with large meals or large amounts of any one food. In the laboratory, IBS patients have exaggerated responses to a meal, supporting the notion that the IBS gut is hypersensitive (see below). This may engender the belief that particular foods 'cause' the disease, and create food aversions that are the result of IBS, not its cause. There is no compelling evidence for specific food allergy or 'sensitivity' in IBS. Nevertheless, certain food components with demonstrable gut effects can aggravate the symptoms (see Chapter 6, Dietary advice).

A motility disorder?

Irritable bowel syndrome has long been thought of as a motility disorder, a view supported by the typically chaotic bowel habit. Certainly intestinal transit is abnormal in many patients. In some, transit is slow (true constipation), in others it is fast (true diarrhea) and, in the textbook case, fast and slow transit alternate. As a group, IBS patients have excessively variable transit time. This is why their stools tend to vary in kind from lumpy to watery and why the timing of their bowel movements tends to be chaotically irregular. Laboratory workers have claimed to find other motility abnormalities, including aberrant electrical activity, but these have not been confirmed.

A neurohumoral disorder?

One concept that has survived the motility era is that the fault lies in the nervous control of the intestine rather than in the intestine itself. Over the last half-century much research has focused on the nervous plexuses found in the wall of the intestine, now called the enteric nervous system (ENS). Often referred to as the 'gut brain', the ENS contains as many neurons as the spinal cord. The study of the ENS and its connections with the CNS (Figure 3.1) has spawned a new discipline, neurogastroenterology. Its devotees believe that the answer to IBS lies in understanding the physiology and chemistry of the ENS. The system is certainly complex and has many analogies with the CNS. For example, it contains most of the neurotransmitters found in the CNS. During sleep, the electrical rhythms of the intestine occur at the same

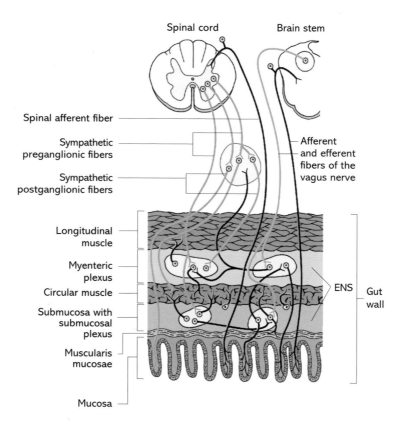

Figure 3.1 The enteric nervous system (ENS) and its connections with the CNS. Descending pathways from the higher centers in the brain are believed to modulate the activity of afferent visceral pathways carrying sensory information from the gut. This may provide a mechanism whereby psychological factors (e.g. expectation, mood and attention) could influence the intensity of visceral symptoms and of gut reactions to stimulation.

rate as those of the brain, and patients with IBS tend to have abnormal REM sleep.

Cholinergic receptors were once seen as critical. They were considered a promising site of pharmacological intervention because gut spasm was thought to underlie the pain of IBS. Few believe this now, and interest these days is focused on the gut serotonin receptors, which are involved in gut motility and secretion and probably visceral pain perception. The gut is extraordinarily rich in serotonin. Other candidates are opiate, cholecystokinin and α-adrenergic receptors. While drugs acting at these sites may relieve some symptoms in some IBS patients, the complexity of the ENS and its receptors makes it unlikely that a single malfunctioning neurohumoral interface explains the whole syndrome in every case.

An inflammatory disorder?

Up to 25% of IBS patients relate the onset of their IBS to an attack of gastroenteritis. Persistent symptoms after such an illness are more likely after a bacterial than a viral infection and after a longer than a shorter illness. Does a low-grade inflammatory response persist after the infection has gone? The discovery in diarrhea-prone IBS patients of intraepithelial lymphocytes and CD25 +ve T-cells has been cited as evidence of persistent infection and immune activation. However, these were not typical IBS cases (they were selected on suspicion of having inflammatory bowel disease), and changes in the gut epithelium fail to explain the malfunctioning gut musculature. In another study, colon biopsies from unselected IBS patients were indistinguishable from controls when interpreted blind by two pathologists. Admittedly, low-grade inflammation could be sub-cellular, perhaps involving inflammatory mediators. However, this is yet to be demonstrated in unselected IBS patients or to occur where it matters most – in the ENS and its muscular connections.

The colon is 'the dark continent' of the GI tract and the principal residence of the gut flora. Despite the extraordinary diversity of these organisms and their vast interface with the gut we know little of their role in health and disease. To be sure, pathogens cause recognized gut diseases, and gnotobiotic (germ-free) rats are unhealthy rats, but could any gut organism play a role in a disorder of gut function such as IBS? It is a fashionable idea, but difficult to prove. Some proponents of the inflammation theory for IBS attribute the inflammation to a harmful change in gut flora, and are studying treatment with probiotics. Probiotics are preparations of living organisms whose metabolism has potentially beneficial features, especially lactobacillus and bifidobacteria. Ingested in sufficient numbers, they repopulate the lower gut and, thereby, are believed to exert various health benefits. These are speculations, but certain probiotics have been successful in the treatment of childhood reovirus infection and show promise in traveler's diarrhea and even Crohn's disease. Their use in IBS is currently the subject of basic research and clinical trials. Meanwhile, health-food stores already sell a wide variety of probiotic preparations.

A psychological disorder?

Numerous studies have demonstrated psychological morbidity and a history of abuse in patients referred to academic institutions. Moreover, it is certain that psychological factors intensify IBS symptoms. Hence there is a widespread belief that IBS has a psychological origin. However, if psychosocial morbidity is a feature of IBS why is it absent in those with IBS in the community who do not seek help? One must take care to distinguish the psychosocial profile of IBS sufferers in general from that of the minority who are referred to specialists. One must manage the whole person, to be sure, but it is wrong to assume psychosocial morbidity in every patient and to do so can be deeply resented.

A hypersensitive gut?

During the 1980s, the idea grew that IBS is essentially a sensory abnormality. As a group, IBS subjects were known to have intestines that overreacted to environmental stimuli such as stress, eating and drugs. When the rectum or sigmoid was distended by inflating a balloon, patients with IBS reported discomfort or pain at lower volumes or pressures than normal controls. Low pain thresholds were also found in the small intestine and even the esophagus. On the other hand, somatic pain thresholds in the same patients were normal or even high. This remarkable difference led to the concept of 'visceral hypersensitivity'. This is a neat idea that explains many of the clinical features of IBS, especially the unpleasant feelings that patients report. It implies that abnormal motor activity is a reflex reaction – an irritable organ overreacting to normal stimuli. But what makes the intestine more sensitive? An attack of gastroenteritis appears to do so in the 30% of sufferers who go on to have IBS. In addition, psychological status may be important. Stressful life events often precede the onset (or, at least, the reporting) of IBS symptoms. Also, in the laboratory, some people can make their gut more sensitive by thinking about it and less sensitive by relaxing deeply.

The visceral hypersensitivity story is an appealing one as it can embrace other hypotheses. (It can, incidentally, provide doctors with a tidy framework to explain IBS to patients and can also help them convince patients that they should avoid aggravating factors such as caffeine, stressful confrontations and certain drugs.) However, the story is not perfect. In the lab, some IBS patients fail to say 'ouch' when the balloon is blown up in their bowel, while the rectum is not particularly sensitive in people with rectal symptoms, such as feelings of incomplete evacuation. Will visceral hypersensitivity be the dominant IBS hypothesis a decade from now? We are not sure.

An abnormality of gut–brain interaction?

Related to the visceral hypersensitivity hypothesis is the notion that the abnormality in IBS lies in the interaction between a person's gut and their brain. This theory embraces psychological as well as physical factors and respects the indivisibility of mind and body. It fits comfortably with the proposed biopsychosocial model of disease or, rather, of the person with the disease.

Positron emission tomography (PET), a sophisticated new way of detecting activity in the brain, has recently been used to show that in normal people, when the rectum is distended, a particular part of the brain lights up – the anterior cingulate gyrus (Figure 3.2). In a small group of IBS patients, this has failed to happen and a different part of the brain has lit up – the left prefrontal cortex. Functional magnetic resonance imaging and other technologies have been employed with similar results. The number of patients studied in this way is small, but the findings have attracted much interest. One interpretation is that descending pathways that inhibit gut sensory transmission are less active in IBS (Figure 3.1). The clinical significance of these findings remains uncertain. One suggestion is that the experience of IBS (or consulting about IBS) is partly a matter of the way people feel and think about the sensations they get from their intestines.

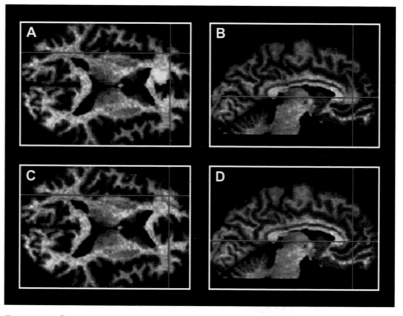

Figure 3.2 Brain imaging techniques illustrate changes in cerebral blood flow and presumably neural activity in response to a stimulus. This early example shows activity in the anterior cingulate cortex in response to the gut stimulus, in this case rectal distension, in a control subject (upper images). In an IBS subject (lower images) the cingulate is not active, but there is increased activity in the prefrontal cortex. Could the anterior cingulate cortex serve as a control switch retarding noxious signals in normal people, while its failure to do so in IBS subjects lets such signals through to the conscious mind? These and similar small observational studies permit speculation, but no definitive conclusions. Certainly science is now acknowledging the gut–brain interaction long recognized by clinicians. Reprinted from Silverman et al. 1997, with permission of Elsevier Science.

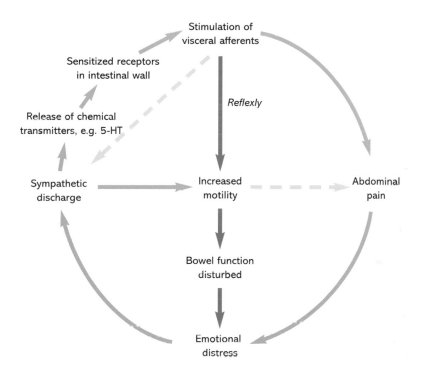

Figure 3.3 A model of IBS emphasizing the role of the sensitive gut and showing one way in which an emotional reaction to the symptoms might perpetuate them, setting up a vicious cycle. Other models and other mechanisms have been proposed.

Thoughts, feelings and vicious cycles

Does emotional distress cause IBS? Expert opinion is divided. There is no doubt that strong emotion can disturb intestinal function acutely. The child who gets a stomach ache when it is time to go to school, the student who has to rush to the toilet before an exam, the young wife whose abdomen swells and hurts when her mother-in-law comes to stay, all demonstrate the fact that the gut reacts to stress. There are also many banal reasons why bowel habit might be disturbed: travel (especially across time zones), other changes in routine, unwise fast foods, bingeing on food or drink, inadequate or unpleasant toilet

31

facilities, weight-reducing diets, menstrual periods, pregnancy, antibiotics, analgesics and many other drugs.

Does a person's mental state cause gut symptoms to persist? It is hard to prove. There are certainly different ways in which a person can react to a bowel upset or a bellyache. They can shrug it off as a temporary nuisance and quickly forget it ever happened. Or they can panic, fearing a serious disease like colitis or cancer, but be too embarrassed to tell anyone about it. If they do get upset – and lower gut symptoms are peculiarly upsetting, being unpleasant, mysterious and embarrassing – then their anxiety may exacerbate the symptoms and cause them to persist. Anxiety activates the sympathetic nervous system and, as demonstrated experimentally, this makes the gut more sensitive. So a vicious cycle might arise with bowel symptoms and anxiety exacerbating each other (Figure 3.3). A scenario like this could explain the results of a study of people suffering a bad attack of acute gastroenteritis. While these previously well people were recovering in hospital, they were assessed psychologically. They were then followed up to see who would have continuing bowel symptoms diagnosable as IBS. These turned out to be the people who had been most unwell in hospital and also those who had scored highest for anxiety and somatization, that is, the worriers and the body-conscious. However, the conclusion that gut infection causes IBS mainly in psychologically susceptible individuals is weakened by the absence of premorbid data. Did these people have IBS before their infection? Was their anxiety and somatization already there or was it induced by their hospitalization? Such questions illustrate the difficulty in assigning an etiology for IBS. Of every hypothesis, one has to ask 'Are the candidate phenomena cause or effect, or just coincidence?'

Reporting bias. A disease like IBS, which consists of subjective symptoms, is liable to reporting bias. This may occur with the reaction to experimental interventions or in patients' attitudes towards their symptoms and the circumstances of their lives. An example of the former follows. If a volunteer having a balloon inflated in the rectum knows it might cause pain, he or she is more likely to report pain; thus apparent hypersensitivity might really be heightened expectation of pain. When this bias is avoided by doing big and small inflations and sham inflations in random order so that the subject cannot guess what is coming next, IBS patients do not, after all, feel the balloon at lower volumes than normal. Rather, they tend to report any rectal sensation as unpleasant, even painful. It seems that they expect pain and so they get it.

Patients' attitudes towards their symptoms may be displayed in many other ways. A series of hospital IBS patients were asked to look at a collection of words, some of which were unpleasant or negative, and to memorize them. The words they remembered best were the unpleasant ones. Moreover, they thought they had been shown unpleasant words that they had not. The medical counterpart of this negative mindset is a tendency to attach serious significance to symptoms, even transient ones.

This pessimistic attitude may not be relevant to intestinal misbehavior in the first place, but it is certainly a feature of people who complain to doctors about their intestinal symptoms. Doctors in a general practice in Hampshire, UK, compared patients who had consulted them for IBS with people in their practice who had the same symptoms but had not consulted. One main difference they found was that consulters harbored fears of serious disease more than non-consulters. (See also Table 3.1.)

TABLE 3.1

Consulters with IBS compared with non-consulters

- Increased number of symptoms
- Apparently increased symptom severity
- Pain more prominent
- Greater psychosocial morbidity
- Increased healthcare-seeking behavior
- Increased neuroticism, tendency to somatize
- Heightened fear of serious disease (see Table 5.1, page 52)

Causes and mechanisms – Key points

- IBS has no known cause or structural manifestation.
- Pathogenesis is also unknown, but hypotheses based on diet, motility, ENS dysfunction, inflammation and psychopathology all have advocates.
- Visceral hypersensitivity embraces most other hypotheses and can help patients to understand current knowledge.
- Research observations in IBS patients may represent coincidence or epiphenomena.

Key references

Aziz Q, Thompson DG. Brain–gut axis in health and disease. *Gastroenterology* 1998;114:559–78.

Collins SM. A case for an immunologic basis for irritable bowel syndrome. *Gastroenterology* 2002; 122:2078–80.

Gorard DA, Farthing MJG. Intestinal motor function in irritable bowel syndrome. *Dig Dis* 1994;12:72–84.

Gwee KA, Graham JC, McKendrick MW et al. Psychometric scores and persistence of irritable bowel after infectious diarrhoea. *Lancet* 1996; 347:150–3.

Mayer EA. Breaking down the functional and organic paradigm. *Curr Opin Gastroenterol* 1996; 12:3–7.

McKee DP, Quigley EMM. Intestinal motility in irritable bowel syndrome: is IBS a motility disorder? Part 1. Definition of IBS and colon motility. *Dig Dis Sci* 1993;38:1761–72.

McIntosh D, Thompson WG, Patel D, et al. Is rectal biopsy necessary in irritable bowel syndrome? *Am J Gastroenterol* 1992; 87:1407–9.

Naliboff BD, Munakata J, Fullerton S et al. Evidence for two distinct perceptual alterations in irritable bowel syndrome. *Gut* 1997;41: 505–12.

Silverman DHS, Munakata JA, Ennes H et al. Regional cerebral activity in normal and pathological perception of visceral pain. *Gastroenterology* 1997;112:64–72.

Talley NJ, Spiller R. Irritable bowel syndrome: a little understood organic disease. *Lancet* 2002;360:555–64.

Thompson WG. Probiotics for irritable bowel syndrome: a light in the darkness? *Eur J Gastroenterol Hepatol* 2001;13:1135–6.

Whitehead WE. Psychosocial aspects of functional gastrointestinal disorders. *Gastroenterol Clin N Am* 1996;25:21–34.

The secret of successful management of IBS is to recognize it quickly and confidently. The importance of positively identifying the syndrome cannot be exaggerated. Many primary care doctors don't make diagnoses. Pressed for time, perhaps, they move directly from complaint to treatment. However, unless they make a clear diagnosis, doctors are not in a position to provide the education, reassurance and prognosis the patient wants and needs. If the doctor says only that nothing is wrong, some patients will conclude, resentfully, that the doctor 'thinks it's all in my head'.

Diagnosis is made from the history. At first sight, this is difficult because there is no single, uniform presentation. The trick is to find out if the presenting symptom is accompanied by others which, taken together, tell us firstly that the problem is with the intestine and secondly that the problem is likely to be a disorder of function rather than structure. To achieve this, physicians need to know the words and phrases that patients use for these symptoms, as well as the correct definition of each symptom. This chapter suggests good questions to ask in order to help make an IBS diagnosis.

The symptoms of IBS

There are three categories of IBS symptoms:

- abdominal pain or discomfort
- disordered defecation and rectal symptoms
- abdominal bloating or distension.

All three are represented in the Manning diagnostic criteria for IBS (Table 1.1, page 10, and Table 4.1), but the Manning criteria have largely been superseded by the Rome II criteria (Table 1.4, page 13, and Tables 4.1 and 4.2), which are practical and simple to use. Two of the three Rome II criteria (in the absence of 'alarm' symptoms or physical findings) are sufficient to make a diagnosis of IBS. The symptoms comprising the criteria require further analysis if confidence in this diagnosis is to be achieved, and are examined below.

TABLE 4.1

Manning criteria and their interpretation

Symptom	Meaning
Abdominal pains lessen after defecation*	The pains come from the lower intestine
When there are pains, the stools are more frequent*	Intestinal function is altered
When there are pains, the stools are looser*	Intestinal function is altered
Bloating or distension (increasing through the day)	The condition is probably non-organic
Rectal feelings of incomplete emptying	The rectum is irritable
Passage of mucus per rectum	The rectum is irritated

* The first three Manning criteria are the Rome II criteria, and two of the three are necessary to link the pain to altered bowel habit and diagnose IBS (in the absence of physical findings and alarm symptoms)

Abdominal pain or discomfort. Pain from the intestine can vary from a twinge or an ache to terrifying agony. Some women describe it as worse than being in labor. Many IBS patients are admitted to surgical wards as 'possible acute abdomen', only to be discharged when the pain settles down, the surgeon's diagnosis being couched in vague terms like 'non-specific abdominal pain' or 'pelvic pain'. The pain is usually in the abdomen but not necessarily so. It can be felt anywhere between the nipples and the thighs, front or back. However, it usually betrays its intestinal origin by the connections between it and defecation, as all the criteria remind us (Tables 4.1 and 4.2). Typically, it eases off after defecation but sometimes it worsens. Usually, the change in bowel habit that occurs when the pains begin is towards more frequent and looser stools, but sometimes it is towards less frequent and harder stools. IBS pain is usually different from that of structural disease. It can be very brief, in 'stabs' lasting a few seconds, and it is often diffuse. Attacks of pain can vary greatly in severity, in character and in location, whereas the pains of structural disease tend to be stereotyped. Pain from IBS

TABLE 4.2

Questions designed to elicit the Rome II criteria*

In the last three months, did you often have discomfort or pain in your abdomen?*

If 'yes':

- Does your discomfort or pain get better or stop after you have a bowel movement?

- When the discomfort or pain started, did you have a change in the usual number of bowel movements? (Either more or fewer?)

- When the discomfort or pain started, did you have either softer or harder stools?

If two of the above three symptoms are present and alarm symptoms and signs are absent the diagnosis is IBS.

* The Rome II criteria (Table 1.4, page 13) specify '12 weeks or more in the past 12 months…'; the 3-month period used here is more suitable to clinical use
Adapted from the modular questionnaire in: Drossman DA, Corazziari E, Talley NJ, et al. *The Functional Gastrointestinal Disorders*, 2nd edn. McLean (VA): Degnon, 2000:678

often goes away for weeks or months at a time, sometimes during times of relaxation, like holidays.

When the pain is in the upper abdomen and when, as often happens, it also worsens after food, it is frequently labeled 'dyspepsia', which leads to fruitless endoscopies. This error is easily avoided by using the Rome II IBS criteria, which, by relating the pain to defecation, localize the problem to the intestine.

Patients with IBS sometimes turn up in urology clinics as 'possible ureteric colic' and, particularly, in gynecology clinics, where lower abdominal pain is labeled 'pelvic pain'. This label is unfortunate because unnecessary laparoscopy or hysterectomy is liable to ensue.

Seldom is the pain of IBS truly colicky, coming and going in cycles of a few minutes, as in intestinal obstruction. Nor is it continuous day and night. Such relentless pain is either due to malignant disease (particularly of the pancreas) or it is functional pain. Functional abdominal pain is a distinct entity (see Tables 1.2 and 1.3, pages 11 and 12), having no features to link the pain to the intestine or to any other organ. It can develop in an IBS patient but it is more intransigent than IBS, like other chronic pain syndromes.

Disordered defecation and rectal symptoms. Bowel symptoms are a troublesome part of IBS but are liable not to be elicited accurately. Most people are embarrassed to talk about defecation and stools, which have been described as society's last taboo. Patients use euphemisms and circumlocutions that have to be decoded. The doctor's temptation to skimp this part of the history should be resisted. Bowel symptoms are often the ones that bother the patient most and must be taken seriously.

Disordered defecation. Three interviewing tips help doctors understand disordered defecation.

- Keep asking questions until it is understood what the patient means when they say, for example, 'I'm dreadfully constipated' or 'I keep needing to go'.
- Ask about the form or appearance of the stools as well as the frequency of defecation to avoid misdiagnosing constipation and diarrhea. Some patients with IBS do have true constipation and/or true diarrhea, sometimes intermittent, sometimes alternating. It is seldom constant. The bowel habit is often misinterpreted. The key question is whether the stool is lumpy (pellety), which implies slow intestinal transit, or liquid/runny, which implies fast transit. It saves time and embarrassment to show the patient illustrations or a printed scale that uses everyday language to describe stools in seven categories that reflect their transit time (Figure 4.1).
- Ask about previous bowel habit as well as the present one so that a change to looser and more frequent stools is not overlooked. This change can appear to the patient as the spontaneous (and welcome) relief of constipation, in which case it may not be volunteered.

Rectal symptoms trouble some patients with IBS more than does abdominal pain or bloating. The feeling of incomplete evacuation (sometimes called 'rectal dissatisfaction') can be troublesome. *Urgency of defecation* is defined as excessively strong calls to stool or as urges to open the bowel that make the patient rush to the toilet. Urgency can be disabling, especially when associated with frequent defecation, as is

Stool form	Appearance	Type
Separate hard lumps, like nuts (hard to pass). Result of slow transit		1
Sausage-shaped but lumpy		2
Like a sausage but with cracks on its surface		3
Like a sausage or snake – smooth and soft		4
Soft blobs with clear-cut edges (easy to pass)		5
Fluffy pieces with ragged edges, a mushy stool		6
Watery, no solid pieces. Result of very fast transit		7

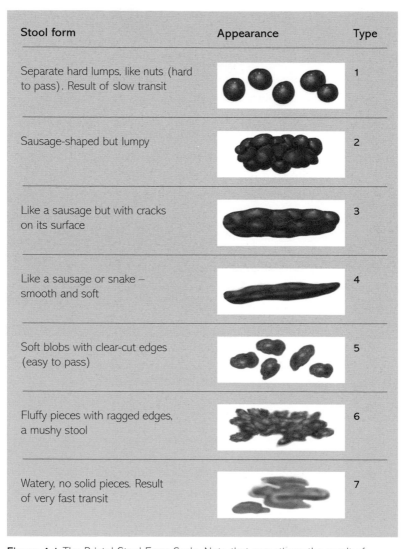

Figure 4.1 The Bristol Stool Form Scale. Note that sometimes the result of defecation consists of more than one stool type, in which case the 'slower' type is the first to be passed. Types 1 and 2 occur in true constipation (Latin 'constipare', to crowd or press together). Types 6 and 7 constitute true diarrhea (liquid stools). Type 4 is the ideal as it is the type of stool whose passage is least often associated with discomfort or effort. People vary a lot in the type of stool they pass, but this variability is exaggerated with IBS. From Heaton et al. 1991.

often the case in the early morning ('the morning rush hour'). There is an analogy with the symptoms of an irritable bladder (sometimes called 'detrusor instability') in which the sufferer has repeated urges to pass small amounts of urine. Urgency of defecation can lead to incontinence of feces. This is a very distressing symptom, even if the soiling is minor, but it is one that patients seldom volunteer as it makes them feel embarrassed or ashamed of themselves. Even without incontinence, urgency can destroy patients' social lives, their sexual relationships, and even their careers. These symptoms are intermittent. Constant frequency, urgency or incontinence are probably not due to IBS.

Unproductive calls to stool or 'want to but can't' is another symptom of an irritable rectum, and is also seldom volunteered. It is common and annoying and can generate a constant awareness of the rectum. Do not confuse this feeling or the feeling of incomplete evacuation with *tenesmus*. Tenesmus is a violent and painful urge to defecate, which occurs in proctitis and other ulcerating diseases of the rectum, but rarely in IBS.

Pseudodiarrhea and pseudoconstipation. The symptoms of an irritable rectum convince many patients that they have diarrhea or constipation when they don't – their stools are of normal form and consistency. This is called pseudodiarrhea when there is predominant urgency and frequency, and pseudoconstipation when fruitless straining occurs due to excessive awareness of the rectum. The way to distinguish these from true diarrhea and constipation is to ask about the form of the stools. Better still, get the patient to keep a record of each defecation for a week or so, noting the form of each stool as well as the date and time of its passage (Figure 4.2). The distinction is not an academic one; prescribing an inappropriate laxative or antidiarrheal agent will earn the doctor no thanks!

Some IBS patients notice the passage of *mucus* with their stool, but it seems to occur much less often than reported by previous generations.

Abdominal bloating or distension is a very common symptom in IBS and occasionally the dominant one. The bloating is often visible to the patient and their partner. Women are more likely than men to experience this symptom. Many are asked if they are pregnant and

Bowel record card

Please record the type of stool you pass each time you go to the toilet and bring this card with you next time you see the doctor. To decide which stool type you have passed, refer to the description below the chart. If a stool is partly one type, partly another, write down both numbers.

Date	Time	Stool type (number)

Type 1 Separate hard lumps, like nuts (hard to pass)
Type 2 Sausage-shaped but lumpy
Type 3 Like a sausage but with cracks on its surface
Type 4 Like a sausage or snake – smooth and soft
Type 5 Soft blobs with clear-cut edges (easy to pass)
Type 6 Fluffy pieces with ragged edges, a mushy stool
Type 7 Watery, no solid pieces

Figure 4.2 A bowel record form for patients to fill in for their doctor.

some claim to feel as if they are. Because the symptom is not common in men, it is omitted from the Rome II criteria.

Bloating is never constant and unremitting; indeed, it can come and go within minutes. It is absent on waking and characteristically worsens as the day goes on so that, in the evening, sufferers loosen or change their clothing. A patient may claim that the distension never goes away but, on examination, it turns out that what bothers her is a lower abdominal fat pad!

Patients often call the sensation of bloating 'trapped wind' or 'gas', but intestinal gas volume is not altered. Nevertheless, laboratory experiments show gastrointestinal gas to be handled and perceived abnormally by bloated patients, especially after fat ingestion. Many believe they are passing excessive flatus but, in most cases, they are not. Other gas symptoms are gurglings or rumblings (technically called 'borborygmi'), and these may occur without bloating.

Non-intestinal symptoms. In specialist practice at least, patients with IBS often complain of other unexplained symptoms, especially from the upper gut and urinary tract. These non-intestinal symptoms are common in themselves, and a true relationship to IBS is unproven. Unlike the linkage between abdominal pain and bowel disorder, they are not useful as diagnostic criteria. They are probably less common in mild cases. The concomitance of IBS and these seemingly unrelated symptoms in referred patients may be a pointer to somatization and psychosocial problems.

Upper gut symptoms include:

- heartburn
- excessive fullness after meals
- nausea.

Less commonly, there is globus sensation ('lump in the throat') or esophageal discomfort on swallowing (odynophagia), easily mislabeled dysphagia. These are the symptoms of an irritable pharynx, an irritable esophagus and, in the case of nausea, an irritable stomach, respectively, and their occurrence reminds us that, in many patients, the problem is not just an irritable bowel but an irritable gut.

Non-intestinal symptoms include fatigue, probably the most common and, in referred patients, sometimes the most troublesome symptom. *Urinary symptoms* tend to be urgency and frequency of urination, but there may also be feelings of incomplete emptying. Urodynamic tests show these patients to have an *irritable bladder*. Women commonly experience *dyspareunia*.

Muscular aches and tenderness can be widespread and lead rheumatologists to diagnose fibromyalgia syndrome; a more appropriate label might be 'irritable muscles'. *Backache* and *headache* are common complaints in patients with IBS.

How to diagnose IBS

Irritable bowel syndrome, like migraine, depression, and even angina, is diagnosed primarily by the pattern of symptoms. Questions eliciting the Rome II criteria (Table 1.4, page 13, and Table 4.2) lead to diagnosis, provided physical signs or alarm symptoms are absent (Table 4.3). Tables 1.4 and 4.4 indicate symptoms whose presence increases

TABLE 4.3

Some 'alarm' symptoms and signs suggesting structural gut disease

- Rectal bleeding
- Weight loss*
- Continuous diarrhea
- Recent onset of constant distension
- Anemia
- Fever
- Family history of colorectal cancer, IBD, celiac disease
- Areas with endemic gut disease (e.g. *Giardia lamblia*)

* Occasionally IBS patients lose weight because they reduce food intake to avoid meal-induced symptoms

confidence in an IBS diagnosis and reminds us of key historical features. The more of the symptoms in Table 1.4 that are present, the more likely is the diagnosis to be IBS (see Figure 1.1, page 10). The Rome I and II criteria select similar subjects and are specific and reasonably sensitive for IBS. However, like any test, symptom criteria must be used thoughtfully. Doctors should be on the watch for alarm symptoms and

TABLE 4.4

Key historical features of IBS

- Multiple symptoms
- Variable and intermittent symptoms
- Pain with intestinal features
- Altered defecation
  - frequency
  - form (Figure 4.1)
  - passage (urgency, straining, feeling of incomplete evacuation)
- Abdominal bloating/distension, particularly if intermittent (more common in women)
- Absence of alarm symptoms (Table 4.3)

take into account particular risks of organic disease (e.g. giardiasis in endemic areas, lactose intolerance in non-caucasians, or a family history of colon cancer, inflammatory bowel disease or celiac disease).

Table 4.2 indicates the questions to ask in order to elicit the Rome II criteria. These questions determine the presence of abdominal pain and uncover 'intestinal' (i.e. defecation-related) features of the pain. Tables 4.5–4.7 illustrate some helpful and unhelpful questions to ask patients in order to better understand their pain, abnormal bowel habit and bloating.

Possible physical signs of IBS have not been scientifically investigated for their diagnostic value. However, many patients have abdominal tenderness. It is often said to be over the colon, but the position of the transverse and sigmoid colon is so variable that, in practice, the

TABLE 4.5

Helpful and unhelpful questions about pain

Helpful

- Is the pain always in the same place or does it move around? (Often the latter is true in IBS.)
- How often do you get it? (IBS pain can be surprisingly occasional.)
- How long does it last each time you get it? (It can be surprisingly short-lived.)
- What happens to the pain when you have your bowels open or pass wind or gas from the back passage? (Usually it eases, but not necessarily.)
- If you are having a trying or worrying time, are you more likely to get the pain?

Unhelpful

- Does it come on or worsen after food? (Any pain from the digestive system can do this, including IBS.)
- How bad is it? (IBS pain can be trivial or excruciating.)
- What does it feel like? (Qualitative assessments are too subjective to be useful; adjectives like 'stabbing' are meaningless.)
- Does it come on at night? (Contrary to popular belief, IBS pain can do this.)

TABLE 4.6

Helpful and unhelpful questions to ask about bowel function

Helpful

- What was your bowel habit before all this started?
- How many times do you 'go' on a good day/a bad day?
- Do you have to rush to the toilet?
- Have you ever failed to get there in time and soiled your pants?
- Does the stool run out of you like water? (True diarrhea.)
- When you have been to the toilet, do you feel as if you have not emptied yourself properly, as if there is still something inside?
- Do you sometimes feel the need to go but there is nothing there to pass?
- Do you have to hold your breath and push for a long time?
- Do you see mucus, slime or clear jelly-like material on the stool?

Unhelpful

- Are your bowels regular? (Too vague!)
- Do you get constipated? (Too vague!)
- Do you get diarrhea? (Too vague!)

TABLE 4.7

Helpful questions to ask about bloating and distension

- Does your tummy ever feel swollen or bloated?
- Is it ever visibly swollen so that other people notice?
- Is the distension there when you wake up in the morning? (If 'yes', it's not IBS.)
- Is it worse at any particular time of day?
- Is it better or worse in the evening?

tenderness can be anywhere. The anal canal too may be tender on digital examination. Obviously, an abdominal mass or enlarged organ cannot be explained by IBS and requires investigation.

Differential diagnosis. The presence of the Rome criteria together with the absence of alarm symptoms and of physical findings indicate that IBS is the likely diagnosis. However, each one of the symptoms of IBS can have a structural cause, even a serious one.

In Western countries, the most important structural diseases causing abdominal pain and/or altered bowel habit are colon cancer, inflammatory bowel disease and celiac disease. These are common, so physicians should keep them in mind as they question and examine patients. Colon diverticula do not account for IBS symptoms despite the earlier belief that they have a similar cause. Persistent diarrhea or constipation can represent functional disorders, but these have their own diagnostic criteria (and different therapeutic procedures). To put IBS into a practical context, Figure 4.3 illustrates how often different gut diseases are encountered by family doctors.

IBS symptoms are not those of cancer but, of course, two such common diseases sometimes coexist. For this reason, and this reason alone, we recommend that patients over 50 years of age should undergo a colonoscopy. (For that matter, any first-degree relative of a

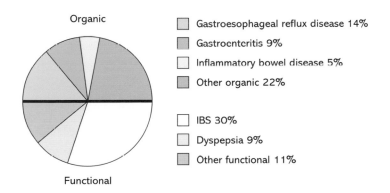

Figure 4.3 Among 3111 adult patients consulting their general practitioner, 255 (8.3%) had a gut problem. The figure shows the distribution of the diagnoses in these patients determined by a panel that reviewed the case records 6 months after the consultation. Note that half the patients had a disorder of gastrointestinal function and 30% (2% of all the 3111 screened patients) had IBS. From Thompson et al. 2000.

person with colon cancer or a previous colon polyp – whether or not they have IBS – should have a colon examination by the age of 50. In the USA, some even recommend colonoscopy for all people at age 50.)

Careful history and physical examination including anal inspection seldom misses a diagnosis of inflammatory bowel disease (IBD). A family history of IBD should prompt a gut investigation. There is no evidence that a short delay in diagnosing subclinical IBD is harmful, provided that the doctor follows up carefully. IBS may occur together with IBD, and the symptoms of an IBD patient should be monitored to ensure that treatment is appropriate.

It has been suggested that many cases of IBS are due to lactose intolerance or celiac disease. However, these and similar proposals come from studies of biased patient samples by researchers with special interests. Accounting for all these possibilities is expensive. To be sure doctors should be aware of IBS patients at risk for these disorders (e.g. non-caucasian milk lovers, persons from endemic celiac areas such as Ireland or northern England), but automatic testing for every possibility is unworthy of, and may even detract from, a thoughtful doctor–patient encounter.

Before adopting celiac immunological screening (or any other screening test) in every IBS patient, we must know if the research data apply generally, and whether clinical clues such as family history or anemia do not indicate celiac risk more cost-effectively. (Is the prevalence of IBS in celiac patients any more than that in the general population? We suspect not.)

Investigations

Often, no investigations are needed. If the history is typical, the patient is young, and there is a clear relation to stress or dietary change, it is meddlesome to do any tests. Carrying out tests could even be counterproductive, raising doubts in the patient's mind about the functional diagnosis and creating anxiety that can take a long time to allay.

Many physicians recommend some routine screening tests such as a blood count, C-reactive protein or erythrocyte sedimentation rate.

However, for this very common disease, rote testing adds to the cost with no evidence of increased diagnostic accuracy. Most patients in British family practice get no tests.

Absolute indications for many tests are really indications for referral to a gastroenterologist, namely, any of the alarm symptoms included in Table 4.3, or suspicion of the diseases discussed in the previous section. A relative indication is a short or atypical history.

Few family physicians perform sigmoidoscopy (about 10% in the UK and Canada). Thus, insistence on sigmoidoscopy as part of a routine IBS work-up would involve specialists in every case, which is impractical. We firmly believe that IBS is usually best managed in primary care. In fact, there is increasing evidence that endoscopy is of little diagnostic value in typical cases. If it is done and the insufflation of air reproduces the patient's pain, he or she may be helped to understand and accept an explanation of the problem along such lines as: 'This demonstrates that at least some of your pain is coming from the lower bowel. Since the lower bowel is healthy – I know it is because I have looked at it – the fact that it hurt when it was stretched means that it has become oversensitive or irritable.'

Gut motility tests and tests for gut hypersensitivity are research tools and have little diagnostic value in IBS. Imaging studies of the intestine are not routinely required. Their indication depends upon the risks and clinical suspicion discussed under differential diagnosis.

Diagnosis – Key points

- IBS can be diagnosed only by symptoms.
- Key symptoms are abdominal pain, altered and unpredictable bowel habit and bloating.
- The more symptoms are present, the more likely is IBS.
- Detailed bowel history is essential, including stool form.
- Few if any tests are required, depending upon clinical circumstances.
- Beware alarm symptoms and signs.

Clinical circumstances determine other tests. Where giardiasis is endemic it may coexist with an irritable bowel. In older patients, one should be alert to cancers such as those of small bowel or ovary.

Key references

Camilleri M, Delgado-Aros S. Much to do about gas. *Gastroenterology* 2002;123:933–4.

Delvaux M. Do we need to perform rectal distension tests to diagnose IBS in clinical practice? *Gastroenterology* 2002;122:2075–8.

Heaton KW, Ghosh S, Braddon FEM. How bad are the symptoms and bowel dysfunction of patients with the irritable bowel syndrome? A prospective, controlled study with emphasis on stool form. *Gut* 1991; 32:73–9.

Kruis W, Thieme CH, Weinzierl M et al. A diagnostic score for the irritable bowel syndrome. Its value in the exclusion of organic disease. *Gastroenterology* 1984;87:1–7.

Manning AP, Thompson WG, Heaton KW et al. Towards positive diagnosis of the irritable bowel. *BMJ* 1978;2:653–4.

Pearson DJ. Pseudo food allergy. *BMJ* 1986;292:221–2.

Pignone M, Rich M, Teutsch SM et al. Screening for colorectal cancer in adults of eaverage risk: a summary of the evidence for the US Preventative Health Services Task Force. *Ann Int Med* 2002;137:132–41.

Sanders D, Carter MJ, Hurlstone DP et al. Association of adult coeliac disease with irritable bowel syndrome: a case-controlled study in patients fulfilling Rome II criteria referred to secondary care. *Lancet* 2001;358:1504–8.

Talley NJ, Phillips SF, Melton LJ et al. Diagnostic value of the Manning Criteria in irritable bowel syndrome. *Gut* 1990;31:77–81.

Tibble JA, Sigthorrson G, Foster R et al. Use of surrogate markers of inflammation and Rome criteria to distinguish organic from non-organic intestinal disease. *Gastroenterology* 2002;123:450–60.

Thompson WG. Irritable bowel syndrome and coeliac disease (letter). *Lancet* 2002; 359:1346.

Thompson WG. Gastrointestinal symptoms in the irritable bowel compared with peptic ulcer and inflammatory bowel disease. *Gut* 1984;25:1089–92.

Thompson WG, Heaton KW, Smyth T, Smyth C. Irritable bowel syndrome in general practice: prevalence, management and referral. *Gut* 2000;46:78–82.

Thompson WG, Longstreth GF, Drossman DA et al. Functional bowel disease and functional abdominal pain. *Gut* 1999;45(suppl II):II43–7.

Vanner SJ, Depew WT, Patterson WG et al. Predictive value of the Rome criteria for diagnosing irritable bowel syndrome. *Am J Gastroenterol* 1999;94:2912–17.

In the previous chapter, we outlined how IBS can be diagnosed promptly and confidently in most cases. This is the bedrock of good management. Only with a confident diagnosis can the doctor reassure the patient effectively, but reassurance is not always effective. In a study of IBS patients attending English general practitioners, we found that more than half the patients waiting to see the doctor harbored fears of serious disease and, unfortunately, most patients still had this fear after seeing the doctor (Table 5.1). We believe this was due to lack of diagnostic confidence in the doctor because when, in a separate study, we asked GPs why they referred patients to specialists, they gave as their principal reason 'diagnostic uncertainty'. The previous chapter of this book is aimed at helping doctors (and ultimately patients) avoid such uncertainty.

Explaining the diagnosis

Once the doctor is reasonably confident of the diagnosis, the patient should be told what is wrong, and the doctor should state categorically that the symptoms are not those of cancer or other serious disease. It is also important to find out the patient's beliefs about their symptoms

TABLE 5.1

Disease fears in primary care patients just before seeing the doctor

	Percentage of patients with IBS* (n = 76)	Percentage of patients with organic disease (n = 100)
Fear of cancer	46	30 (vs IBS p < 0.04)
Fear of other disease	9	10
Total with fears	55	40 (vs IBS p < 0.05)

* Disappointingly but importantly, only 29% of IBS patients had lost their fears after visiting their family doctor

and to correct any misconceptions, stressing that IBS does not increase the risk of developing any other disease. If tests have revealed colon diverticula, their lack of relevance should be explained: half of elderly Westerners have such diverticula and nearly all are asymptomatic; very few develop diverticulitis.

This good news should be tempered with a realistic prognosis: the doctor can point out that IBS symptoms tend to be chronic, or to recur throughout life (Figures 2.4 and 2.5, pages 19, 20). Hopes of permanent cure are unrealistic and likely to be dashed by recurrence. Unless warned of this, patients may consult other doctors and undergo unnecessary and even dangerous tests and treatments. Of course, a diagnosis of IBS confers no immunity to other gut disease, which occurs as often in IBS patients as in the general population. Alert physicians will detect alarm symptoms, risk indicators and physical findings.

Reassurance alone is not enough. Some explanation of IBS must be given too, and it must be tailored to the patient's level of understanding. It may be helpful to describe the gut as 'touchy' or excitable, so that it overreacts to everyday experiences such as stress, eating and defecation, or to gut stimulants such as caffeine, laxatives and drugs. This explanation is in accord with the 'visceral hypersensitivity' hypothesis outlined in Chapter 3 (Causes and mechanisms). Some doctors liken IBS to a headache – a nuisance rather than a disease. It may be a big nuisance, but it causes no physical damage.

Aggravating factors

Patient and doctor together should review the patient's lifestyle in search of aggravating factors. Questions about working hours and family commitments can be very revealing. Some patients seem never to relax. Others suspect and eliminate foods, but individual foods are seldom guilty. More likely to disrupt gut function than any specific food are irregular and rushed meals, such as occur with shift work, business lunches, or just in busy households.

Patients with diarrhea as their main symptom should be told about the laxative effects of sorbitol, the artificial sweetener in many sugar-free gums, jams and sweets/candy. These effects are not well known. In contrast, most people who believe they are lactose intolerant are not (at least if they are caucasian) and, even if they are, can cope with modest amounts of milk without getting symptoms (Chapter 6, Dietary advice).

Drugs must not be forgotten – many disturb gut function, causing abdominal bloating and pain as unwanted side-effects (Table 5.2). Obviously, moderation should be advised with tobacco, alcohol and caffeine. In addition to its damaging effect on lungs and heart, tobacco can also provoke gut motility.

Doctors can also help patients learn to cope with difficulties such as precipitate bowel movements, social events with unknown toilet facilities, or unsanitary public toilets – often the bane of the IBS patient's existence.

TABLE 5.2

Some drugs that commonly disturb bowel function

Drugs causing constipation

- Opiates (e.g. codeine, morphine)
- Phenothiazines (e.g. chlorpromazine)
- Tricyclic antidepressants (e.g. amitriptyline)
- 5-HT$_3$ antagonists (e.g. ondansetron, alosetron; see Chapter 7)
- Calcium channel blockers
- Anticholinergics
- Calcium carbonate

Drugs causing diarrhea

- Misoprostol
- 5-HT$_4$ agonists (tegaserod, see Chapter 7)
- Antacids containing magnesium hydroxide
- Herbal teas containing senna
- Alcohol
- Caffeine
- Sorbitol (see Chapter 6)

Other agendas and psychosocial aspects

At an early stage, the doctor should search for unspoken agendas. Gut symptoms may be a vehicle for seeking care, more socially acceptable than psychological symptoms, yet psychosocial disturbances often underlie a person's decision to consult the doctor. A distressing event such as bereavement, separation from a loved one, or loss of employment may enhance an individual's awareness of their body and its sensations and prompt them to seek healthcare. A simple example is the death of a parent from colon cancer, in which case explaining that the patient's symptoms are not those of cancer may be the only therapy required. At the other end of the complexity spectrum, sexual or physical abuse or family disintegration can demand the assistance of a skilled counselor. Some patients who have coped with IBS for years lose their ability to do so when they develop anxiety, depression or panic.

A more tricky issue is secondary gain. For example, IBS symptoms may be used to influence family members. A clue to this may be excessively concerned behavior on the part of the person accompanying the patient to the doctor. In this situation the doctor must tread carefully as, in a curious way, some relationships are nourished by illness in one partner. The patient who believes that their symptoms entitle them to a disability pension poses another special dilemma. The symptoms are unlikely to improve until the claim is settled, yet a disability pension is hardly an encouragement to better coping. In such cases, to avoid conflict of interest, the decision about disability should be delegated elsewhere. IBS can be difficult enough to manage when these confounding issues are recognized, impossible if they are not.

Alternative treatments

Up to one third of IBS patients seek alternative or complementary therapies. These paramedical treatments are increasingly popular even though their rationale, methods and content are often mysterious, and few have been submitted to scientific inquiry. Although none is of proven efficacy in IBS, they are usually harmless and may succeed by exploiting the placebo response. Doctors should take note of their patients' alternative therapies, not necessarily to criticize them, but rather to guard against harm from them, particularly from radical diets and exorbitantly priced 'supplements'. In lieu of regulatory surveillance, physicians may turn to sources such as www.quackwatch.com.

The caring relationship

Few current measures improve a patient's symptoms beyond the placebo effect. This effect must not be dismissed, for it can be substantial. In a randomized, placebo-controlled trial of a drug for the treatment of IBS (Figure 5.1), the improvement in the placebo arm was

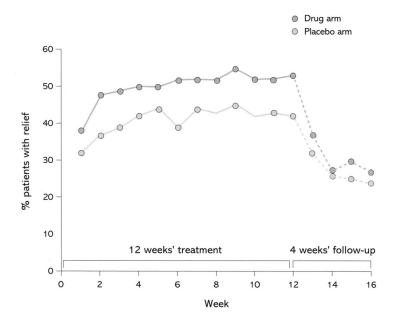

Figure 5.1 Typical results of a randomized, placebo-controlled trial of a drug in the treatment of IBS illustrating the components of a therapeutic response. The difference between the number relieved of symptoms in the drug and placebo arms is the *therapeutic* gain. The trial shows the drug to be effective significantly more often than placebo. The magnitude of the gain, 10–12%, seems superficially disappointing. However, it is similar to the therapeutic gains of other accredited drugs such as the H_2-receptor antagonists in healing peptic ulcers. Note the improvement in the placebo arm (about 40%). Note also that when the drug and placebo are discontinued, the number of patients with relief of symptoms drops dramatically, but not to zero.

about 40%. When the drug and placebo were discontinued, the number of patients with relief of symptoms dropped dramatically, but not to zero. The drop may represent the loss of the placebo effect and of the therapeutic gain in the drug arm. Since the natural history of IBS involves fluctuating symptoms, the end-of-trial improvement over baseline (about 25%) may be what the situation would have been if no treatment had been given. These two influences (placebo effect and natural remission) are at work in every successful therapeutic encounter. Obviously, these powerful improvement tendencies are present in subjects given the test drug as well. Indeed, were a drug's benefit limited to the therapeutic gain of 10–12%, its clinical value would be doubtful. Doctors instinctively utilize these helpful assets, the likelihood of natural improvement and the force of their therapeutic personality, to coax maximum benefit from treatment. The natural history of a disease (except when downhill as in terminal cancer) and the placebo effect are exploited in every successful treatment, and in IBS they may be the most powerful of all.

The lesson to be learned from this is the therapeutic power of a relationship with a healthcare provider. Such a relationship is most effective when it involves an empathetic doctor and includes a firm diagnosis, careful discussion of possible causes, and a clear, convincing explanation of the nature of IBS. This approach is time-consuming at first, but it soon pays a dividend (Figure 5.2). It seems that in an IBS patient, what matters is *how* a doctor diagnoses, reassures, educates and empathizes. When the doctor proffers treatment, how it is given is more important than its nature.

The doctor should take pride in minimizing tests, therapies and referrals. In most cases, we believe this can be achieved without trivializing the symptoms or denying their disrupting effects. The ultimate goal should be a patient who perceives their symptoms as a manageable nuisance and rejoins that silent majority of people with IBS who have learned to cope and do not seek healthcare.

Follow-up

One follow-up visit is advisable to confirm that the diagnosis is secure and that the patient understands it. That visit satisfies many patients,

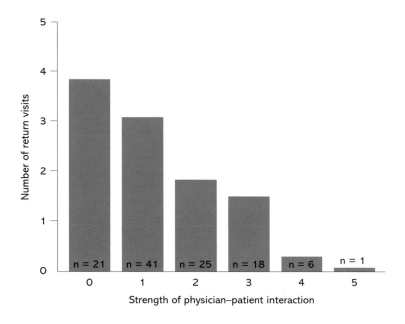

Figure 5.2 Findings from a retrospective look at the case notes of 112 IBS patients followed up at the Mayo Clinic, USA. The number of return visits was inversely proportional to the strength of the physician–patient interaction at the first visit. This interaction was scored according to comments in the notes indicating that a psychosocial history was obtained and that a personalized discussion took place. Reproduced with permission from Owens DM et al. *Ann Intern Medicine* 1995;122:107–12.

but others need continuing care by a family doctor. Every visit should include sympathetic listening and careful questioning about new symptoms. Do not repeat investigations unless there is a clear indication. To do so undermines patients' confidence in the diagnosis and is costly. Patients with social and psychiatric problems unresponsive to treatment need ongoing access to a physician, perhaps with the assistance of a mental health professional (see Chapter 8, Psychological treatment).

Approach to treatment – Key points

- Firm diagnosis is essential to successful management.
- Physicians should address patients' fears and provide a realistic prognosis.
- A strong therapeutic relationship and maximization of the placebo effect is important.
- A patient's agenda (often unstated) should direct management.

Key references

Kruis W, Thieme CH, Weinzierl M et al. A diagnostic score for the irritable bowel syndrome. Its value in the exclusion of organic disease. *Gastroenterology* 1984;87:1–7.

Owens DM, Nelson DK, Talley NJ. The irritable bowel syndrome: long term prognosis and the patient–physician interaction. *Ann Intern Med* 1995;122:107–12.

Patterson WG, Thompson WG, Vanner SJ et al. and the IBS consensus conference participants. Recommendations for the management of irritable bowel syndrome in family practice. *Can Med Assoc J* 1999;161:154–60.

Suarez FL, Savaiano DA, Levitt MD. A comparison of symptoms after the consumption of milk or lactose-hydrolyzed milk by people with self-reported severe lactose intolerance. *N Engl J Med* 1995;333:1–4.

Talley NJ, Phillips SF, Melton LJ et al. Diagnostic value of the Manning criteria in irritable bowel syndrome. *Gut* 1990;31:77–81.

Thompson WG. Management of the irritable bowel syndrome. *Aliment Pharmacol Ther* 2002;16:1395–406.

Thompson WG, Hungin APS, Neri M et al. The management of the irritable bowel syndrome: a European primary and secondary care collaboration. *Eur J Gastroenterol Hepatol* 2001;13:933–9.

Thompson WG. Placebos: a review of the placebo response. *Am J Gastroenterol* 2000;95:1637–43.

Thompson WG, Heaton KW, Smyth T, Smyth C. Irritable bowel syndrome in general practice: prevalence, management and referral. *Gut* 2000;46:78–82.

Thompson WG, Heaton KW, Smyth GT, Smyth C. Irritable bowel syndrome: the view from general practice. *Eur J Gastroenterol Hepatol* 1997;9:689–92.

Thompson WG. Gastrointestinal symptoms in the irritable bowel compared with peptic ulcer and inflammatory bowel disease. *Gut* 1984;25:1089–92.

The scientific evidence for a role of diet in the treatment of IBS is weak. This does not mean there is no place for dietary advice. Patients expect it and even demand it, and there are common-sense reasons for responding (Table 6.1).

Meal-related symptoms

In many patients, eating provokes abdominal pain or a violent urge to pass stool. If the stool is loose, the patient may think the food has 'gone straight through'. The doctor should explain to the patient that this is the manifestation of a normal physiological phenomenon – postprandial peristalsis of the large intestine or a 'mass movement' – and that, since their bowel is sensitive, the reaction is exaggerated. When the gut overreacts in this way, what matters is not so much what is eaten as how much is eaten. Big meals, particularly fatty ones, should be avoided. Fat delays stomach emptying and impairs the movement of gas through the intestine. Reducing meal size and fat content may have an incidental benefit; that is, it may help the patient who wants to lose weight. Another thing to point out is that rushed or stress-filled meals may impair digestion.

Diet history or record

Being poorly trained in nutrition and dietetics, doctors are often reluctant to get involved, but a brief dietary history (Table 6.2) or a 5–7-day diet record can reveal obvious problem areas. Not eating breakfast may help to explain constipation, as may a diet devoid of fruit and vegetables. A high coffee intake not only stimulates the gut directly, but may also contribute to nervous tension and consequent gut irritability. Diarrhea can be caused or exacerbated by a high intake of fiber-rich foods or products, or of products sweetened with fructose or sorbitol (Table 6.3). The same can be true of beer and, particularly in non-caucasians who lack adequate amounts of the enzyme lactase, milk and other dairy products. Research suggests, however, that lactose in

TABLE 6.1

Reasons for giving dietary advice

- Many patients expect such advice.
- Eating provokes symptoms in many patients, so 'diet must matter'.
- Dietary discussion has a placebo effect, and shows the doctor cares.
- Dietary discussion is an opportunity to promote healthy eating habits.
- Some food products can aggravate IBS symptoms.

TABLE 6.2

Questions to ask in a brief dietary history

- What do you have for breakfast?
- How many cups of coffee (or tea or cola drinks) a day do you drink?
- How much gum, preservatives or sweets/candy do you consume daily? (Table 6.3)
- How often do you eat fruit/vegetables?
- What kind of bread do you eat and how many slices a day?
- How much milk do you drink?
- Is there any food you avoid? If so, why?

moderate doses, as in a glass of milk, does not trigger IBS symptoms even in subjects with proven lactose malabsorption.

Elimination diet for specific food intolerances

Specialists disagree about the importance of specific food intolerances in IBS. This is partly because it is difficult to do research in this area and good scientific data are scanty. Patients are sometimes convinced from past experiences that they react to specific foods. Such food intolerances can have a psychological basis (food aversion). This can be distinguished from physical food intolerance, but to do so with certainty requires up to eight double-blind challenge tests. This is impractical and rarely, if ever, done. Meanwhile, we suggest the following pragmatic approach where food intolerance is suspected.

TABLE 6.3

Foods and drugs containing fructose and sorbitol

Excessive ingestion of fructose or sorbitol may cause diarrhea, thereby aggravating IBS

	Fructose (g/100 g)*	Sorbitol (g/100 g)*
Fruit		
Cherries	7.2	12.6
Grapes	10.5	
Pear juice	20	12
Dates	31	
Honey and jams		
Honey	40.5	
Quince jelly	20.6	27.2
Jams	4.5	25.6
Soft drinks		
Cola	6	
Lemon	5.3	
Orange	5.6	
Confectionery		
Chocolate	42.4	
Chewing gum		59.3
Vanilla ice cream		81.3
Drugs		
Antacids		5
Bronchodilators		5
Expectorants		5.7
Miscellaneous		
Multivitamins		8

* Maximum values

- Consider physical food intolerance only if the patient has true diarrhea (liquid stools) at least part of the time.
- If the diarrhea is occasional, get the patient to keep simultaneous food and bowel records (see Figure 4.2, page 42) for a period long enough to include at least two episodes of diarrhea. A likely dietary culprit is a food or drink that preceded every episode, provided there were few or no instances when it was consumed with impunity.
- If the diarrhea is constant or nearly so, and there is no obvious excess of fiber, caffeine, sorbitol or fructose consumption, the diagnosis is unlikely to be IBS. Such a patient needs referral to a gastroenterologist. After ruling out other causes of diarrhea the gastroenterologist may consider sending them to a dietitian for help with an elimination diet.

If the patient has an aversion to a non-essential food, like garlic or a single vegetable, he or she need not be persuaded to eat it. However, the physician should intervene if avoidance of food seems to threaten nutritional status.

Bran and high-fiber diets

Wheat bran has long been popular in the treatment of IBS, but its apparent success in an early controlled trial was not confirmed. Some specialist-referred patients who are already taking bran are advised to try stopping it, and half of them seem to benefit from doing so. It may be that bran usage is so widespread in primary care that patients referred to hospital are mostly 'bran failures'. Symptoms that are said to worsen on bran are diarrhea, abdominal pain and bloating.

Patients who are most likely to improve on bran are those whose bowel habit tends towards constipation (lumpy stools). In general, fiber or fiber supplements do help constipation. Therefore, in constipated IBS patients, if a brief dietary history or a 5–7-day diet record shows infrequent use of fiber-rich foods, and provided the patient is motivated to change their eating habits, we recommend a naturally fiber-rich diet. This should emphasize breakfast as a meal where it is easy, convenient and pleasant to eat a lot of wheat fiber because this is the most laxative type of dietary fiber. It is possible that the benefits of this approach are partly from placebo effect and from the general improvement in health that can follow a switch to a better diet, but these are benefits worth having.

Constipated patients who are not motivated to change their eating habits, or who cannot take in enough fiber-rich foods to cure their constipation, may benefit from wheat bran, particularly the raw, coarse flaky variety, which has the strongest laxative effect (Table 6.4). This can be washed down with water or fruit juice, or be mixed with suitable foods like breakfast cereals, yogurt and thick soups. The dose should start at one tablespoonful a day and increase if necessary, or until side-effects occur. The amount consumed should be monitored by referring to stool form and the need to strain rather than by frequency of defecation. A simple stool record may be helpful (see Figure 4.2). If wheat bran is not tolerated, there are several pharmaceutical bulking agents available, such as ispaghula or psyllium preparations (Table 6.4).

TABLE 6.4

Bran and other bulking agents

Agent	Availability	Comments
Wheat bran (raw, 'natural' bran)	Health-food shops, pharmacies	Coarse, flaky variety is most effective
Cooked bran products	Food shops (e.g. bran-based breakfast cereals, bran muffins)	Probably less effective but more palatable
Wheat fiber concentrate	Pharmacies (prescription and OTC)	In convenient sachets
Ispaghula/psyllium*	Pharmacies (prescription and OTC)	Granulated or powdered, some flavored
Sterculia gum*	Pharmacies (prescription and OTC)	
Methylcellulose	Pharmacies (prescription and OTC)	

* These products swell greatly when wetted so need to be taken with plenty of fluid to avoid possible bolus obstruction
OTC, over the counter

There is no sanctioned 'IBS diet'. However, the internet and other media propose various diets for bowel disease, often with much hype. Most such diets are harmless as well as valueless, but some have potential for harm. If the patient feels better on a media-derived diet (presumably because of placebo effect) the doctor need not interfere. Nevertheless, the diet should be enquired about so that advice can be given if the diet seems nutritionally inadequate.

Dietary advice – Key points

- Patients with IBS expect dietary advice.
- There is no authenticated 'IBS diet'.
- Adequate dietary fiber may prevent constipation.
- Patients should moderate their intake of foods that 'irritate' their gut, such as caffeine, alcohol, sorbitol and fat.

Key references

Fernandez-Banares F, Esteve-Pardo M, De Leon R et al. Sugar malabsorption in functional bowel disease: clinical implications. *Am J Gastroenterol* 1993;88:2044–50.

Fowlie S, Eastwood MA, Prescott R. Irritable bowel syndrome: assessment of psychological disturbance and its influence on the response to fibre supplementation. *J Psychosom Res* 1992;36:175–80.

Hammonds R, Whorwell P. The role of fibre in IBS. *Int J Gastroenterol* 1997;10:9–12.

Nanda R, James R, Smith H et al. Food intolerance and the irritable bowel syndrome. *Gut* 1989;30:1099–104.

Thompson WG. Doubts about bran. *Lancet* 1993;344:3.

Thompson WG. Management of the irritable bowel syndrome. *Aliment Pharmacol Ther* 2002;16:1395–406.

'Not a single study has been published that provides compelling evidence that any therapeutic agent is efficacious in the global treatment of IBS.'

K.B. Klein 1988

Nowadays physicians are supposed to practice 'evidence-based' medicine. However, practicing doctors know that little evidence underlies most therapeutic decisions. Much of their daily work consists of reacting to myriad clinical problems based on their experience, on their knowledge of physiology, psychology, pathology etc., and on their skills in handling patients – educating, encouraging and consoling; that is, in practicing the 'art' of medicine. Without this amalgam of science, art and instinct, medicine would not exist. Until half a century ago physicians had little to offer beyond the placebo effect and the natural tendency of most diseases to remit. So it is still with IBS. Klein's oft-quoted lament (above) has held true. A survey covering IBS treatment trials from 1987 to 2000 came to a similar conclusion. This failure to prove efficacy for any drug had many explanations.

- Published trials had design flaws, such as imprecise entry criteria, too few subjects, improper randomization and blinding, short duration, the use of crossover design, and inappropriate statistics.
- There is a profound placebo response to any IBS treatment (Table 7.1; Figure 5.1, page 56). Drossman noticed this was greatest when the drugs were dispensed by a doctor (which surely says something about the healing power of a caring relationship). It has been claimed that it is difficult for a trial drug to show benefit in IBS because of the high placebo response, but this response is also high in peptic ulcer trials.
- The pharmacological targets of therapy may be inappropriate since there is no known pathogenesis upon which to base them. In fact, treatments are directed at symptoms.

- For 200 years colon spasm was thought to underlie IBS symptoms, and until recently IBS was known as the *spastic colon*. This theory is unsubstantiated and now widely doubted; yet the notion lingers that drugs that relax gut smooth muscle should relieve the symptoms. Drugs to counter gut spasm (i.e. those with anticholinergic/antimuscarinic properties, such as atropine and the quaternary ammonium synthetics) have been used since the 1940s with no convincing evidence that they are effective.
- The new drugs being tested are aimed at the enteric nervous system (ENS, see Chapter 3, Causes and mechanisms). But the ENS is thought to be as complex as the brain itself. It is far from certain

TABLE 7.1

Patients responding to placebo in some clinical trials

	Trial substance	Placebo responders (%)
For IBS		
Lichstein 1967	Belladonna	30
Wayne 1969	Librax	38
Søltoft 1975	Bran	69
Fielding 1980	Trimebutine	88
Fielding 1982	Domperidone	57
Lucey 1987	Bran	71
Camilleri 1999	Alosetron	40 (approx)
Müller-Lissner 2001	Tegaserod	30
For peptic ulcer*		
	Antacid	55
	Cimetidine	38
	Prostaglandins	44
	Omeprazole	27

* From Thompson WG. *The Ulcer Story*. New York: Perseus Books Group, 1994:344

that, among its myriad receptors and neurotransmitters, or its neural connections with the brain, there lies a single key to the understanding and cure of IBS. To the authors, the chance of developing a 'magic bullet' seems remote.

- Up till now, the subjects for drug trials have been recruited in university centers where the patients have been selected for referral by other doctors (see Chapter 2, Epidemiology, and Figure 2.6, page 21). Such patients are probably unrepresentative. They tend to have severe psychosocial problems such as abuse, depression or panic, which may bias the results of trials, particularly when quality of life is an outcome measure. We know of no published trials done in primary care, yet it is in primary care that drugs to treat the physical symptoms are most likely to prove their worth.

Were a drug truly effective in this troublesome condition, it would presumably be used all over the world. However, in different countries there is much inconsistency in the drugs that are approved for the treatment of IBS (Table 7.2). This must inspire skepticism about the efficacy of any of them. It must also be borne in mind that many popular drugs have the potential to make matters worse or induce new symptoms. Anticholinergics and antidepressants can produce or worsen constipation, prokinetics can worsen diarrhea, and peppermint oil can induce gastroesophageal reflux.

Meta-analysis

A current medical fashion is to combine all the known trials of a treatment in one statistical analysis in an effort to increase the power of the data to give a definite answer. Early, successful examples of meta-analysis involved homogeneously diseased subjects and a finite end-point, such as death or outcome of premature pregnancy. However, these conditions have hitherto not been met in IBS trials.

For example, in two meta-analyses, trials of heterogeneous smooth-muscle relaxant drugs such as anticholinergics, peppermint oil, opioid antagonists and calcium channel blockers have been combined to make the case that this therapeutic approach is effective. However, as already mentioned, the combined trials are flawed. If trial data are flawed, no amount of pooling can make the conclusions valid. The methodological

TABLE 7.2

Some drugs approved for IBS in five countries*

Generic name	Trade name	Action
Australia		
Dicyclomine	Merbentyl	Anticholinergic
Alverine	Alvercol	Papaverine-like
Hyoscine, atropine (D,L-hyoscyamine), scopolamine (L-hyoscine)	Donnatab	Anticholinergic
Mebeverine	Colofac	Antispasmodic
Peppermint oil	Mintec	Carminative
Canada		
Dicyclomine	Bentylol	Anticholinergic
Propantheline	Pro-banthine	Anticholinergic
Hyoscyamine	Levsin	Anticholinergic
Hyoscyamine, atropine (D,L-hyoscyamine), scopolamine (L-hyoscine)†	Donnatal (also contains phenobarbital)	Anticholinergic
Pinaverium	Dicetel	Calcium channel blocker
Trimebutine	Modulon	Kappa opiate antagonist
Peppermint oil†	Colpermin	Carminative
France		
Prifinium	Riabal	Anticholinergic
Alverine	Spasmaverine	Papaverine-like
Mebeverine	Colopriv	Antispasmodic
Pinaverium	Dicetel	Calcium channel blocker
Trimebutine	Debridat	Kappa opiate antagonist

*None of these are supported by a randomized controlled trial that satisfies the criteria of Klein. Alosetron and tegaserod, which have undergone stricter trials, were approved in some countries in 2002; see Table 7.4

† Withdrawn

TABLE 7.2 (CONTINUED)

UK

Hyoscine	Buscopan	Anticholinergic
Dicyclomine	Merbentyl	Anticholinergic
Alverine	Spasmonal	Antispasmodic from papaverine
Mebeverine	Colofac	Antispasmodic
Peppermint oil	Colpermin, Mintec	Carminative

USA

Dicyclomine	Bentyl	Anticholinergic
Hyoscyamine	Levsin	Anticholinergic
Hyoscyamine, atropine (D,L-hyoscyamine), scopolamine (L-hyoscine)	Donnatal (also contains phenobarbital)	Anticholinergic

errors in the studies analyzed are substantial. The trial entry criteria are seldom stated, and only the most recent studies employ diagnostic criteria. Many trials include subjects without pain, and entry criteria permit inclusion in the meta-analysis if 'at least 51% of subjects had IBS'. None of the trials employ the endpoints recommended by an expert panel. Crossover trials, deemed inappropriate for fluctuating conditions like IBS, are included. The numbers of subjects range from 31 to 288, so that few of the trials have statistical power. The included trials lasted from 3 days to 24 weeks and the intervals and outcome assessments vary greatly.

Fortunately, this sorry state of affairs is improving. Trial design for new IBS drugs has become more sophisticated and entry criteria more standardized, while outcome measures now focus on abdominal pain or a global measure that embraces pain and other symptoms. Nevertheless, like the perfect poem, the perfect clinical trial has yet to appear. Continuing challenges include the selection of subjects from whom the results can be generalized to most patients with IBS, guaranteed double blinding, and selection of the most appropriate outcome measures and periods of treatment.

New drugs

Recently the pharmaceutical industry has adopted more satisfactory trial designs, and regulatory agencies and drug benefit programs have begun to ignore studies that fall below these standards (and so should physicians).

Alosetron, a 5-HT$_3$ antagonist, was the first drug to demonstrate global improvement of IBS symptoms in properly defined patients with IBS, provided they had diarrhea. Unfortunately, the drug had to be withdrawn when some patients receiving it were found to have ischemic colitis or severe constipation. It seems likely that many of these patients had preexisting colitis or pseudodiarrhea (frequent pellety stools) and were inappropriately given the drug. Alosetron will shortly be reintroduced with restrictions in the United States for the treatment of women with IBS who also have diarrhea. In 2002, tegaserod, a 5-HT$_4$ agonist, became available in the USA, Australia, Canada and several other countries (40 in all) for women with IBS who are constipated, and so far its only untoward effect has been diarrhea (as anticipated from the drug's prokinetic properties). These new drugs affect colonic transit time. To avoid many of the untoward events that occurred with the first introduction of alosetron, these new drugs must be used only in accurately diagnosed IBS patients with the appropriate bowel habit.

Manufacturers of both tegaserod and alosetron claim the drugs reduce visceral sensation, and animal experiments indicate that tegaserod inhibits visceral afferent nerves involved in pain sensation. Patients taking either tegaserod or alosetron showed improvement on a global measure that included pain, and also in the secondary outcomes of relief of pain and bloating. (It is unknown whether similar results might be achieved with antidiarrheal or laxative drugs through correction of the predominant bowel dysfunction.)

Although these new drugs show promise for treating IBS with diarrhea and IBS with constipation respectively, they are not cures. It must be kept in mind that benefit from a prescribed drug depends less on what is prescribed than on the quality of the doctor–patient interaction when it is prescribed (see Figure 5.2, page 58).

TABLE 7.3

Examples of drugs for specific complaints

Indication	Drug	Comments
Diarrhea	Loperamide, 1–2 tablets three times daily; for incontinence or as needed for episodes of diarrhea	Antidiarrheal agent, tightens anal sphincter
	Diphenoxylate, 1–2 tablets three times daily as needed for episodes of diarrhea	Antidiarrheal agent
	Cholestyramine, 1 sachet one to four times daily	Binds bile salts malabsorbed from fast small-bowel transit
Constipation	Bran to prevent constipation	Adjust dose to suit individual
	Psyllium/ispaghula husk to prevent constipation	Adjust dose to suit individual
Pain		
– Postprandial	Dicyclomine, 10–20 mg before meals	The gastrocolonic response is partially cholinergically mediated
– Chronic abdominal pain (may not be IBS)	Amitriptyline	Sub-antidepressant dose. Titrate from a low starting dose (e.g. 10 mg at night)

Drugs for specific symptoms

We believe that most people complaining of IBS require no drug and
certainly should not be on a drug for very long periods. No chemical
can replace the measures emphasized in Chapter 5 (Approach to
treatment). Nevertheless, drugs may be useful to control individual IBS
symptoms (Tables 7.3 and 7.4). If a woman has IBS despite other
measures and if her bowel habit is mostly diarrhea, alosetron is
appropriate and, if it is mostly constipation, tegaserod may help.
Bowel habit must be properly assessed, for example using the Bristol
Stool Form Scale (Figure 4.1, page 40). Patients who are troubled by
sudden, unpredictable episodes of diarrhea can benefit from a timely

single dose of an antidiarrheal drug such as loperamide (Imodium) or diphenoxylate (Lomotil), e.g. before they leave home. If stools are hard and pellety, the patient may benefit from a bulking agent such as bran or ispaghula/psyllium (see Chapter 6, Dietary advice).

Extrapolating from the pain literature, many physicians recommend low-dose tricyclic antidepressants for IBS patients with debilitating chronic abdominal pain. However, chronic abdominal pain syndrome

TABLE 7.4

Drugs newly available for the treatment of IBS

Drug	Indication	Comment
Tegaserod (Zelnorm) (6 mg twice daily with meals)	IBS with constipation* in women[†] Reassess in one month Maximum treatment 3 months	A $5HT_4$ agonist with prokinetic effects Aside from reversible diarrhea, it appears safe Available in USA, Canada, Australia and several other countries, but not in the European Union
Alosetron (Lotronex) (1 mg twice daily)	IBS with diarrhea* in women[†] Discontinue if constipation**	A $5HT_3$ antagonist with gut slowing effects. Reports of ischemic colitis and severe constipation. Reintroduced in the US only in 2002 with restrictions**

* Subjects for these studies were selected by the Rome I criteria (see Chapters 1 and 4). The notion of diarrhea-predominant and constipation-predominant IBS (D-IBS and C-IBS) was not embraced by the Rome deliberations. Rather, trial designers made the distinctions to ensure that the patients entered in their trials were suitable in relation to the effect of the drug(s) on gut motility. There is a proposed third type called alternating IBS. Many observers believe that these designations are not stable over the course of the disease and that patients switch from time to time. What is important is to ensure that at the time the drug is introduced, the drug is suitable to the patient's current bowel function (see stool form scale, Figure 4.1, page 40)
† Further studies may find these drugs useful in men, but current data suggest otherwise
** The manufacturer and the US Food and Drug Administration have agreed that, in order to prescribe alosetron, physicians will have to attest that they know how to diagnose and treat IBS, when to use the drug, and how to recognize and report side-effects. Patients will be required to sign an agreement acknowledging the risks of the drug. Pharmacists will be instructed only to fill prescriptions that have a sticker sanctioning the prescriber. Phoned or faxed prescriptions will not be permitted, in an attempt to ensure continuing doctor–patient contact

is not IBS, and trials of antidepressants in IBS suffer design flaws similar to those testing the drugs listed in Table 7.2.

Other products

Practitioners of alternative medicine promote many substances and rituals for the treatment of IBS. Most are harmless, but some are not. Some herbal teas contain laxatives, like senna. Irritable bowel syndrome is not caused by *Candida* so there is no role for antifungal drugs. There is anecdote-based enthusiasm in North America for Beano, an α-galactosidase, in the treatment of 'gas'. This enzyme digests some carbohydrates not processed in the small intestine, thereby denying them to gas-forming organisms. On the other hand, malabsorption is not a feature of IBS, so the use of pancreatic enzymes makes little sense. Dimethylpolysiloxane (Ovol) is a surfactant that breaks up bubbles in the secretions of the upper gut. It is used in some countries for the bloating associated with IBS, but there is little proof that it works.

Some believe that IBS involves inflammatory change attributable to the gut flora (Chapter 3, Causes and mechanisms) and is amenable to probiotic therapy with one of the many possible bacteria such as species of acidophilus (yogurt), lactobacillus, bifidobacteria etc. Probiotics are being studied in a variety of gut disorders including IBS, but as yet no conclusions can be drawn. Currently available probiotics have a short

---

Drug treatment – Key points

- No drugs were proven efficacious before 2002. (Trials were faulty.)
- The placebo effect engendered by a good therapeutic relationship is important to all successful treatments (Table 7.1).
- Some drugs may be dispensed short-term for particular IBS symptoms.
- New 5-HT drugs (tegaserod and alosetron, where available) should be prescribed only to accurately diagnosed IBS patients with the appropriate bowel habit (Table 7.4).

shelf-life and the presence of live bacteria at the point of ingestion is not assured, let alone after exposure to gastric acid.

There is pressing need that all treatments be subjected to the same scientific evaluation and regulatory process as are pharmaceuticals. In the twenty-first century, the argument that 'they can do no harm' is not good enough; nor is the mantra 'lack of proof doesn't mean lack of efficacy'. Not only are alternative treatments not uniformly harmless, but their contents are often a mystery.

Key references

Akehurst R, Kaltenhaler E. Treatment of irritable bowel syndrome: a review of randomized controlled trials. *Gut* 2001;48:272–82.

Camilleri M. Review article: Tegaserod. *Aliment Pharmacol Ther* 2001:15;277–89.

Camilleri M, Mayer EA, Drossman DA et al. Improvement in pain and bowel function in female irritable bowel patients with alosetron, a 5-HT$_3$-receptor antagonist. *Aliment Pharmacol Ther* 1999:13;1149–59.

Camilleri M, Choi M-G. Review article: irritable bowel syndrome. *Aliment Pharmacol Ther* 1997;11:3–15.

Jackson AL, O'Malley PG, Tomkins G et al. Treatment of functional gastrointestinal disorders with antidepressant medications. *Am J Med* 2000;108:65–72.

Klein KB. Controlled treatment trials in the irritable bowel syndrome: a critique. *Gastroenterology* 1988;95:232–41.

Müller-Lissner SA, Fumagalli I, Bardhan KD et al. Tegaserod, a 5-HT$_4$ receptor agonist, relieves symptoms in irritable bowel syndrome patients with abdominal pain, bloating and constipation. *Aliment Pharmacol Ther* 2001;15: 1655–66.

Poynard T, Regimgeau C, Benhamou Y. Meta-analysis of smooth muscle relaxants in the treatment of irritable bowel syndrome. *Aliment Pharmacol Ther* 2001;15:355–61.

Shapiro AK, Shapiro E. *The Powerful Placebo: From Ancient Priest to Modern Physician.* Baltimore: Johns Hopkins Press, 1997.

Talley NJ. Serotoninergic neuro-enteric modulators. *Lancet* 2001; 358:2061–8.

Talley NJ, Nyrén O, Drossman DA et al. The irritable bowel syndrome: toward optimal design of controlled treatment trials. *Gastroenterol Int* 1993;6:189–211.

Thompson WG. Management of the irritable bowel syndrome. *Aliment Pharmacol Ther* 2002;16:1395–406.

Thompson WG. Probiotics for irritable bowel syndrome: a light in the darkness? *Eur J Gastroenterol Hepatol* 2001;13:1135–6.

Informal treatment

In a sense, psychological treatment occurs whenever a patient gains encouragement and mental relief from a consultation. Some patients feel better as soon as they know they do not have cancer. Others are content to discover at last what the term 'IBS' means, or to have their symptoms legitimized as a named disease. All these benefits should flow from the first consultation. Explanation and reassurance can have great power but, to achieve their potential, they must be given in an unhurried, personalized way.

Many patients are dimly aware of a connection with stress and are glad to have this confirmed. Some appreciate the link only when they are asked to think back to what was going on in their lives at the time when the symptoms started to be troublesome. Others are loath to admit they have been psychologically distressed. It may save face if the doctor reminds them that we all have strong feelings and then points out that, if these feelings aren't expressed outwardly – by crying, fighting or fleeing, for example – they do not just evaporate but can be internalized and affect the workings of the body. Everyday language testifies to the fact that emotions can upset the gut (e.g. 'gut feelings', 'gut reactions', 'gut-wrenching experiences'). In other patients, different factors may be at work. Table 8.1 suggests phrases that a doctor can use to help a patient recognize the relevance of psychological factors and Table 8.2 presents some questions that may help to uncover them.

Simple measures of this kind suffice for the great majority of patients with IBS, particularly if they are combined with common-sense advice about lifestyle and eating habits. For example:
• avoid excessive working hours
• allow time for the call to stool before rushing off to work
• avoid big meals and alcoholic binges
• ensure peace and relaxation during meals.

Here we must recall the placebo effect. Some think of this as the power of an inert pill, but an inert pill has no power. Rather, it is the

TABLE 8.1

Phrases to introduce a patient to the possible role of psychological factors

- We may not know what causes IBS but we do know it gets worse when people are under stress or are upset.
- This is especially likely to happen in people who have strong feelings.
- It's especially likely to happen when people don't share their feelings but bottle them up inside.
- Some of us express our feelings through our guts, so people talk about 'gut reactions' and 'gut-wrenching experiences'.
- Having gut symptoms is a stress in itself, especially if you don't tell anyone about them.
- Getting upset can make symptoms worse, so it's easy to get into a vicious circle.

TABLE 8.2

Questions to find out whether psychological factors are involved

- What do you think is causing your tummy/bowel problem?
- Does it come on or get worse when you are stressed/under pressure/upset/worried?
- What was happening in your life when the symptoms began to trouble you?
- Do the symptoms make you worried/angry/disgusted?
- Do you show your feelings or do you bottle them up inside?
- Are you always on the go, always 'on edge'?
- What do you do to relax?

pill-giver's behavior that exerts the placebo effect. We believe that this effect should be maximized, and the general measures suggested throughout this book work to this end. The enthusiasm, authority and care with which the instructions or pill are dispensed are crucial. The doctor is the placebo!

The more difficult patient. Some patients do not respond to these simple measures. They may have troublesome relationships at home or at work, excessive responsibilities, or other life situations that are 'hard to stomach' or hard to escape. Some are habitual somatizers or hypochondriacs. Others have been abused as children or suffered some other deprivation that has impaired their ability to cope. Still others have treatable psychiatric disease. All can be offered help and support. This may take the form of a regular visit to the doctor every 1–3 months to review symptoms and treatments and discuss the patient's current worries. Patient advocacy and support groups have done much to increase public understanding and acceptance of IBS, and should help reduce the fears and isolation that many patients feel. Some patients turn to the internet or to alternative practitioners. Doctors may wish to exploit the patient resources listed at the end of this book.

Especially difficult patients are those who take offence at any mention of psychological factors and are convinced that a physical cause for their symptoms will be found if only the right test is done. These patients can sensibly be referred to a gastroenterologist, but the referral letter should make it clear that what is being looked for is not more investigation but authoritative explanation and reassurance.

Of course, not everyone with IBS has a serious psychological problem. Indeed, sufferers who don't consult doctors have no more problems than people without the symptoms. Patients who are referred to academic centers and some others may have significant psychological comorbidity that hinders their ability to cope with physical symptoms. These are patients who consult repeatedly, and not always for IBS. Their symptoms are unlikely to improve until the emotional or mood disorder improves.

Formal psychological treatments

Expert psychological treatment is occasionally necessary, even in primary care settings. Obvious indications are debilitating psychiatric comorbidity, such as panic attacks, agoraphobia, depression or anxiety state. Some experts feel that the most severe cases of IBS benefit from formal psychological treatment.

Good results have been claimed for several types of psychological treatment. However, interpretation of published trials is difficult. All have been carried out in tertiary care settings and the results are not necessarily applicable to primary or even secondary care. Blinded studies are impossible with psychotherapy. Most trials have involved combinations of treatments, typically including relaxation training. A recent review by an expert team concluded that no single treatment is best and that the patient's motivation to have treatment and the therapist's enthusiasm are what matters.

Psychological treatments are not universally available. In the UK, gut-directed hypnotherapy has a following, whereas in North America relaxation therapy, cognitive behavioral therapy and supportive psychotherapy are often advocated (Table 8.3).

Cognitive–behavioral therapy (CBT). Specially trained therapists work to uncover patients' misperceptions of their illness and train them to see their symptoms as less disabling. Positive aspects of IBS are stressed, such as its lack of mortality or disfigurement. Social functioning and physical activity are encouraged, and illness behavior is discouraged or ignored. In the USA, a large National Institutes of Health (NIH)-sponsored study was completed last year (2002) comparing CBT to 'sympathetic education'. The results (unpublished at the time of going to press) favor CBT for 'moderate to severe' IBS.

Relaxation therapy. Relaxation has many variants including meditation, yoga, biofeedback and programmed tightening and relaxing of muscle groups. Audio- and videotapes are available for patients to self-educate, but some of the more formal measures such as biofeedback require a therapist. Regular physical exercise helps some patients to relax.

Gut-directed hypnotherapy. In the UK, some clinical psychologists offer gut-directed hypnotherapy, but these practitioners are in short supply and seldom funded. A few doctors have had the necessary training, but hypnotherapy is time-consuming, involving multiple sessions. At each session, standard induction of the hypnotic state (a state of heightened suggestibility) is followed by repeated suggestions of peace and warmth

TABLE 8.3

Formal psychological treatments used in IBS

Treatment	Comments
Cognitive–behavioral therapy	• Aims to rectify abnormal illness beliefs and perceptions, to reduce illness behavior, and to increase social and physical activity
Relaxation training	• Can include biofeedback, meditation, yoga (arousal reduction) • Available anywhere • Can be recommended by physicians
Gut-directed hypnotherapy	• Can alter gut sensitivity, reactivity • Limited availability of required special training
Dynamic or analytical psychotherapy	• Requires committed psychiatrist forming close relationship with patient • Expensive and impractical for all but the most troubled patients
Antidepressant drugs	• Low doses may have analgesic effect • Therapeutic doses for depression • May be used by generalist or specialist without referral to a psychiatrist

spreading from a hand on the abdomen together with mental pictures of, for example, a calmly flowing river, ending with standard ego-strengthening suggestions. The patient may learn autohypnosis through audiotapes.

Dynamic or analytic psychotherapy. This time-consuming and costly treatment requires a committed psychiatrist or psychologist. A British study claimed impressive success in 'difficult' IBS patients provided the subjects recognized their psychological difficulties.

> **Psychological treatment – Key points**
>
> - Psychological support begins with the first consultation.
> - Diagnosis, education, reassurance and compassion are essential.
> - With IBS, the manner in which treatment is given is more important than the treatment itself. 'The doctor is the placebo.'
> - Formal psychological treatments, some of which target comorbid psychopathology, are difficult to evaluate. (Do they treat IBS, or do they improve wellbeing and coping ability by treating comorbid psychopathology?)

Psychoactive drugs. Drugs, particularly antidepressants in full therapeutic doses, can have a valuable role when there is frank psychiatric illness. Also, when pain is the dominant symptom, *low doses* of tricyclic antidepressants (but possibly not some newer ones like selective serotonin reuptake inhibitors) may have an analgesic effect. The NIH study mentioned above supports the use of antidepressants in 'moderate-to-severe' IBS, but whether this improves IBS directly, or through ameliorating a depression is moot. Otherwise we doubt the value of psychoactive drugs and discourage their use in routine cases.

Conclusions

There are methodological faults with all published trials of psychological treatment for IBS. It can be argued that some of them are not IBS treatments at all; rather, they aim to improve a patient's wellbeing by reducing comorbid psychopathology. It has even been claimed that these treatments are themselves placebos. Certainly, except for psychoactive drugs, a blinded placebo control is difficult to imagine. One must also doubt the general applicability of trial findings in tertiary-care patients motivated to complete lengthy protocols. At the practical level, few patients are sufficiently ill and disabled to justify the money, time and resource consumption of formal psychotherapies. Most therapies require a psychiatrist or psychologist, but the services of these professionals are seldom available (or may not be covered by the patient's health insurance). In the end, a compassionate physician providing an authoritative and reassuring clinical assessment is the most efficient means to give IBS patients the psychological support they need – the same support needed by any person who feels ill, socially isolated and fearful.

Key references

Psychotherapy: Effective treatment or expensive placebo? *Lancet* 1984;I:83–4.

Brody H. The doctor as therapeutic agent: a placebo effect research agenda. In: Harrington A, ed. *The Placebo Effect*. Cambridge, Mass: Harvard, 1997:77–92.

Clouse RE. Antidepressants for functional gastrointestinal symptoms. *Dig Dis Sci* 1994;39:2352–63.

Creed R, Guthrie E. Psychological treatments of the irritable bowel syndrome. *Gut* 1989;30:1601–9.

Creed F. Relationship between IBS and psychiatric disorder. In: Camilleri M, Spiller RC, eds. *Irritable Bowel Syndrome: Diagnosis and Treatment*. Edinburgh, London: Saunders, 2002:45–54.

Guthrie E, Thompson D. Abdominal pain and functional gastrointestinal disorders. *BMJ* 2002;325:701–3.

Jackson AL, O'Malley PG, Tomkins G et al. Treatment of functional gastrointestinal disorders with antidepressant medications. *Am J Med* 2000;108:65–72.

Owens DM, Nelson DK, Talley NJ. The irritable bowel syndrome: long term prognosis and the patient–physician interaction. *Ann Intern Med* 1995;122:107–112.

Talley NJ, Owen BK, Boyce P et al. Psychological treatments for irritable bowel syndrome: a critique of controlled treatment trials. *Am J Gastroenterol* 1996;91:277–86.

Thompson WG. Management of the irritable bowel syndrome. *Aliment Pharmacol Ther* 2002;16:1395–406.

Toner BB. Cognitive–behavioural treatment of functional somatic syndromes: integrating gender issues. *Cognit Behav Pract* 1994;1:157–178.

Whorwell PJ, Prior A, Colgan SM. Hypnotherapy in severe irritable bowel syndrome: further experience. *Gut* 1987;28:423–5.

The past 25 years have witnessed an explosion of interest in IBS. We have learned that its symptoms are prevalent worldwide, that most people with them do not consult doctors, and that people who do and are referred to specialists are prone to psychosocial problems and to unexplained symptoms in other parts of the body. We have begun to see the wasteful practice of diagnosis by exclusion yield to diagnosis by symptom criteria and absence of 'alarm symptoms'. This has benefited patients and reduced healthcare costs. Twenty-five years ago some hospital doctors disparaged IBS patients as 'crocks' or 'neurotics'. That such attitudes now seem rare is progress as well.

However, there is a long way to go. Needless tests are still done and treatments are still given which are not proven to be better than placebo. Many questions and problems remain to engage researchers in the next quarter-century.

Epidemiology

We need to know why only some people with the symptoms of IBS seek medical advice and why even fewer are referred to specialists. Is it all a matter of somatic and psychological comorbidity? Are coping strategies important? How are they acquired? Those who maintain that psychopathology causes IBS symptoms, as opposed to consulting behavior, need to demonstrate that psychopathology is a feature of IBS everywhere.

We need to understand better the natural history of the disease – how often it remits, how often it recurs, and whether the bowel pattern remains constant over time. Is the practice of subdividing IBS into diarrhea-predominant, constipation-predominant and alternating types valid, and is it useful in guiding management?

Causes and mechanisms

Further study of gut motility is unlikely to increase our understanding of IBS, or lead us to a cause. Some experts believe the key lies in the enteric nervous system (ENS). As discussed earlier (Chapter 3, Causes and mechanisms), the ENS is a complex entity, with neural connections to all levels of the gut and to the spinal cord and brain, operating via multifarious receptors and neurotransmitters.

Currently, there is much speculation about the possibility of specific receptor defects in the ENS–CNS axis amenable to pharmacological intervention. The pharmaceutical industry is pursuing this hypothesis with enthusiasm. Lacking a clear pathophysiological model, the industry is investigating a wide variety of agonists and antagonists to serotonin, muscarinic, cholecystokinin, opioid and other receptors. Proof of efficacy for such an agent requires massive and costly clinical trials. Two drugs acting on the serotonin HT_3 and HT_4 receptors have been released in some countries and seem to benefit some symptoms in some patients. But can a condition as diverse as IBS be reversed by a single chemical substance? We have our doubts. Manipulation of ENS neurotransmitters may produce agents that alter aspects of gut function and sensation but, in terms of *curing* IBS, the longed-for 'magic bullet' may turn out to be a will-o'-the-wisp.

Gut hypersensitivity need not originate in the gut, nor even in the ENS. Indeed, many believe it resides in higher centers in the spinal cord or brain, so that IBS is really the result of disturbed brain–gut interaction. Using complex technology such as positron emission tomography and functional magnetic resonance imaging, researchers have shown gut events in IBS patients to be associated with abnormal brain activity (see Chapter 3), leading to the attractive hypothesis that gut supersensitivity is due to impaired central inhibition of sensation. Further research is needed to tell whether abnormal brain activity is indeed a primary pathological process or merely an epiphenomenon.

Those who believe that inflammation lies behind some or all cases of IBS need to demonstrate its presence in IBS subjects and its absence in carefully matched controls. If anti-inflammatory therapy, with its associated risks, is to be contemplated, a means of identifying those likely to benefit is essential.

Until recently, the notion that the gut flora might participate in the pathogenesis of IBS was ignored. Perhaps inspired by the *Helicobacter pylori* story and by the widespread use of probiotics as alternative treatments in other conditions, researchers are now studying these bacterial preparations scientifically and subjecting them to clinical trials for the treatment of IBS. It is early days, but research into the myriad candidate bacterial species that constitute the gut flora seems likely to continue for years to come.

Research into psychological mechanisms and treatments is also certain to continue. Such research must match the sophistication of physiological studies if psychosomatic (or psychovisceral) theories of IBS are to convince the doubters. One thing cannot be doubted – that mind and body often combine to increase the misery of IBS patients. The prominent psychosocial disorders of the patients who attend academic centers have prompted the development of many psychological interventions, but are these relevant to primary care? Recently completed studies of cognitive behavioral therapy and psychotherapy show them to be helpful in severe IBS, but how useful are they to ordinary cases seen by the family doctor? Do psychological treatments simply help patients put up with their symptoms?

Some fundamental questions haunt us. Could IBS turn out to be a subtle and so far unrecognized organic disease like *Helicobacter pylori* infection, in which wellbeing is sometimes further impaired by depression, anxiety, tragedy, or other psychosocial disturbance? Could IBS even be sometimes organic, sometimes psychologically induced? Is it a disease at all or is it, like tears, just a reaction – albeit an exaggerated one – to a person's physical or social environment?

We must maintain open minds. Most ideas about the putative causes of IBS are no longer new. Researchers need novel ideas as well as better investigative tools. We all should be aware too that how observers view IBS is very much influenced by their own experience and there are many viewpoints.

Diagnosis

The Rome criteria for IBS have become the lingua franca for researchers and clinical trialists and we believe they will prove helpful in diagnosis too. The process that generated them is ongoing and, in late 2004, teams of experts from around the world will reconvene. We hope that the Rome III report (which should be available in 2006) will issue new guidance on the predictive value of alarm symptoms and the validity of IBS subtypes.

Without a physical marker, validation of symptom criteria is difficult. Nevertheless, we need to know more about the reliability of such criteria in clinical practice. Similarly, if any 'routine' tests are proposed, their utility should be demonstrated. Moreover, we need to know if regional or demographic characteristics require special testing.

Treatment

The recent clinical trials establishing efficacy and safety for the two newly approved 5-HT drugs, while not perfect, are a breakthrough in the sense that they represent the first serious attempts to test IBS treatments according to modern standards of randomized, placebo-controlled trials. As therapies, the drugs themselves are a more modest advance. They are palliative rather than curative, and help only women – indeed only women with the appropriate bowel habit. Why are they only effective in women? Which women are most likely to benefit? How long and how often should they be consumed? Are there other ENS receptors whose manipulation might yield even more effective palliation? As long as the cause of IBS is unknown, its ideal drug treatment will continue to elude us. We can expect more trials of ENS-acting drugs and perhaps some that act centrally as well.

We can also expect developments on the psychotherapeutic front. The results of the CBT and psychotherapeutic trials mentioned in the last chapter will stimulate controversy and further research. If psychological treatments are beneficial to some IBS sufferers, how are likely beneficiaries to be selected? How can these treatments be made widely available? Can primary care physicians develop the skills and take the time to manage such treatment? Are 'placebo'-controlled trials feasible with psychological therapy? Should trials of psychological treatment have to meet the same standards of evaluation as regulatory authorities now require of drug trials?

There is growing pressure to scientifically evaluate 'alternative' treatments, because so many IBS patients employ them. We have seen a beginning with small clinical trials of probiotics and reflexology. Also, Chinese herbal medicine was the subject of a small trial (although the contents are not fully known, let alone standardized) and there are ongoing trials of acupuncture and food allergy treatments. Surely these treatments, like pharmaceuticals, must be regulated. Not all are harmless.

Doctors must study and attempt to maximize the benefits of the doctor–patient relationship and of the placebo response. Since the emergence of the healing arts, these have been among medicine's most powerful therapies. Their potency remains, particularly in a chronic, benign condition like IBS.

We believe there are exciting times ahead. Research into IBS has become so intense that improved understanding will surely result, and this could benefit patients with functional problems in other body systems. Meanwhile, today's doctors, like their forefathers, must inform their patients with what scientific understanding is available and support them with empathy and common sense.

Future trends – Key points

- Why do only some people with IBS see doctors?
- Are there really gender differences?
- What is the natural history of IBS?
- Better pathophysiological hypotheses are needed.
- What are the ingredients of a successful therapeutic relationship?
- Future IBS research should embrace primary care.

Useful addresses

Patient resources

IBS Network
Northern General Hospital
Sheffield
S5 7AU
UK
Tel: 0114 261 1531
(answerphone)
helpline Mon–Fri 18.00–20.00:
01543 492192
www.ibsnetwork.org.uk

International Foundation for Functional Gastrointestinal Disorders
PO Box 170864
Milwaukee
WI 53217
USA
Tel: 888 964 2001
www.aboutibs.org
www.iffgd.org

Northwestern Society of Intestinal Research
855 West 12th Avenue
Vancouver, B.C.
V5Z 1M9
Canada
Tel: 866 600 4875
www.badgut.com

Physician resources

Quackwatch
www.quackwatch.com

Medline Plus IBS page
http://www.nlm.nih.gov/medlinepl
us/irritablebowelsyndrome.html

Rome Criteria for IBS
www.romecriteria.org

Medscape Gastroenterology page
www.medscape.com/gastroenterol
ogyhome

Functional Brain Gut Research Group
(special interest section of
American Gastroenterological
Association)
c/o UNC Center for Functional GI
& Motility Disorders
CB #7080
778 Burnett-Womack Building
Chapel Hill, NC 27599-7080
USA
www.unc.edu/depts/fbgrg

Index